A act
I in
Y your
O own
B best
I interest

Five Principles to Live By Because
There is No Future in Staying the Same

By Norman Plovnick, PhD

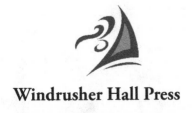

Windrusher Hall Press

International Standard Business Number
978-0-9834336-9-9

Printed and published in the United States of America by
Windrusher Hall Press
P. O. Box 1587
Ponte Vedra Beach, FL 32004

Dedication

To Susan, who always has my back

Contents

PART ONE
ACTING IN YOUR OWN BEST INTEREST (AIYOBI)

PART TWO
WHY BE MORAL

PART THREE
THERE IS NO FUTURE IN STAYING THE SAME

The Search

Ever since I was little, I've been trying to "fix" people. It started with my mother, who was bipolar with a severe anxiety disorder. Sometimes she was crazy manic and took flight for the moon. And then, for months on end, she was hammered by depression and sat woefully in her chair sobbing, angry, depleted, and afraid. As I recall, for a few days a year, she behaved almost normally. My search began. Around age eight or nine, I thought, what can I do to get my mother to behave normally all the time.

The search was fueled by dread and desperation. The darkness had already been wired in, and the scars would remain forever. Nevertheless, the quest began, how to balance the unbalanced and bring peace to the home.

I've never really left that path or mission. Now 74, I have worked in the fields of psychology and neurology all of my life. Half a century ago, I stepped into Manhattan State Hospital with the green ignorance that academic knowledge provides. I was driven to learn and understand so that I could help those poor people. I was hoping to find the answers.

Hopefully, no certainly, I've learned some things along the way. The ideas presented here evolved over five decades of clinical experience, research, personal relationships, and general observations.

Sometimes, I think I've seen it all, and then someone's behavior totally shocks me, and I realize I haven't. So, while my search isn't over, I'm getting close to the end of the line. You know, "knocking on Heaven's door."

I do not belong to any particular school of thought but rather follow the profound theory of common sense. The overriding theme of the book is that if we can act in our own best interest, we can solve many of life's problems. Our most formidable enemy is ourselves. We sabotage ourselves in so many ways. When we engage in self-destructive behavior, we are essentially mentally ill.

The book begins with Five Principles, which are the foundation of the narrative. The profiles of my patients, as well as public figures, reveal how the principles play out in the various stages of life.

In Part One, it is revealed how self-injurious behavior sabotages our well-being, our relationships, and our work. I then explore the clash between irrational emotion and reason and how an inner dialogue can save the day.

In Part Two, I talk about morality and how being moral is in our best interest. Morality is a subject that is often avoided and poorly understood. Our moral behavior and the morality of the people we encounter along the way play an important role in our mental health and well-being.

In Part Three, I explore the challenges faced in adapting to an ever-changing world. Adjusting and adapting to the different stages of life from adolescence to old age is even more demanding. There truly is no future in staying the same.

The book is short, which I always liked. It is a bit preachy and opinionated. You won't agree with everything, but it's honest and contains useful information.

At this point, it has been suggested that I extoll my credentials to win over the trust of the reader. My advice, don't rely on credentials, they can easily be fudged, embellished, and even when accurate, don't mean very much. This is particularly true in health care today, a multi-trillion-dollar industry that uses marketing to lure those hurting and looking for answers. It's the merit of what is being said and done that matters, not the size of the crown of the messenger.

I can tell you about all the degrees and training I have,

the programs I've established, and the broad populations I've served, but I won't. It would take too much time and is really irrelevant. The truth lies in the validity of the message, not who the courier is.

The Five Principles

Here are five principles to live by that will serve us well throughout our lives. They are universal guideposts for growth and problem-solving. I believe we would all be mentally healthier if we were able to employ these principles most of the time. After identifying the Five Principles for you, I'll expand and clarify them even more with examples and personal experiences.

- Act in your own best interest
- Most of the time, you can't control how you feel, but you can control your actions, and if you act in your own best interest, you will feel better
- Make decisions and take action based on reason, not emotion
- What is moral is in our best interest
- There is no future in staying the same

Acting in our own best interest

Whether or not we act in our own best interest is an acid test of our mental health.

When we engage in self-destructive behavior, we are essentially turning against ourselves and, therefore, mentally ill. For what better defines mental illness than engaging in behavior that is detrimental to one's self?

Self-interest doesn't mean being selfish but rather implies behavior that is healthy, productive, and self-enhancing. Acting in our own best interest should be instinctive and readily embraced, and the failure to do so absurd. Nevertheless, we sabotage ourselves all the time. Much in life lies beyond our control, but where we do have control, we often squander it with self-destructive behavior. You can be a genius and still be self-destructive; emotions have a very low IQ.

When we love someone, our goal is to act in their best interest. We are attentive to their well-being and try to facilitate their growth and self-esteem. It doesn't seem that complicated or elusive, yet its execution is daunting. So many of us, children and adults alike, engage in harmful behavior. What is the motive? Why do we do that to ourselves? Is it possible we aren't able to recognize what is in our best interest?

Controlling how you feel

Can we control how we feel? People tell us we can—that you *should* be able to control your feelings. I don't believe we can. Whether we employ positive self-talk, yoga, meditation, therapy, or drugs, it is challenging to change how we feel. How we feel, whether optimistic or pessimistic, is mostly determined by how we are wired. Our genes and neurobiology interacting with early life experiences create neural pathways that shape our feeling states and moods.

How many times have you heard it said that you shouldn't "feel that way?" Best-selling books tell us that we can banish all our negative emotions, whether we feel fearful, discouraged, jealous, or angry by thinking more positively. This kind of advice can be very frustrating, as if we can easily do that on command. "It's your attitude that's the problem," they tell us, "you're making yourself worse."

How we feel is not easily changed. We can't change our nervous system or change who we are and how we emotionally react to life's events. But we can control our behavior, our actions, and if we act in our own best interest, we will feel better.

Reason over emotion

Who is at the helm—reason or emotion? When emotion takes the wheel, we're likely heading for the cliff. Emotionally driven behavior is the primary reason we don't act in our own best interests. At times, our emotions lead us to make bad decisions and act irrationally.

Why are emotions irrational, and why do they have such power over us?

We know emotions have intense psychic energy because when we are in the grip of one, like love, fear, jealousy, and rage, the feeling consumes us. We may also understand that emotions are not logical, and actions stirred by them often end in failure. Nevertheless, they evoke in us behavior that is difficult to control.

The behavior involved in jealousy exemplifies the irrationality and uncontrollability of that emotional state. When we feel jealous and possessive, it's hard to control our actions. The more jealous our behavior, the more we betray ourselves. We know better but undermine ourselves anyway. Instead of holding on to the person, our questions, accusations, neediness, and dependency drive them away.

Establishing a powerful, rational inner-voice is essential

for living well. In our relationships, work, finances, and, most importantly, in our self-appraisal, reason must prevail over feelings.

Why be moral

How do you define morality? For some, morality is strongly linked to religion, but for many others, it means being honest, helpful to others, and employing the concept of fairness. Is being moral beneficial to one's self? In the long run, I'd say it is most definitely beneficial. Good moral conduct yields rewards beyond helping others. It is self-enriching and paves the way to inner peace and elevated self-esteem. You can sleep well when you tell the truth. When we are acting in our own best interest, we are also acting morally.

Superior moral ethics are the antithesis of psychopathy (sociopathy, antisocial personality). Psychopathic behavior is moral behavior at its most depraved. Its gluttonous greed has no bounds. The psychopath's behavior typically results in short-term gratification but long-term implosion. The reckless pursuit of money or power or sex eventually turns into a self-destructive force. Compulsions spin out of control; arrogance, entitlement, and poor judgment take over. While in the grip of narcissistic behavior, the psychopath fails to anticipate the consequences of their actions. Dramatic examples include high profile cases like Jeffrey Epstein, Bernie Madoff, and Harvey Weinstein. I'm never surprised when psychopaths hurt others. The amazing thing is their failure to see how their actions were leading to their self-destruction.

Morality is a personal concept, often described as how you treat others and conduct your life. On the other hand, morality is not about your views on abortion or climate change. The ability to evaluate moral conduct in others is essential to our well-being, and good moral values will guide you in assessing the moral integrity of others.

For centuries, philosophers and ethicists have asked perplexing questions about morality. Are there levels, differences in the quality of moral behavior? Is moral behavior motivated by the fear of "getting caught" or principles of integrity? How do our children learn to be moral? Is moral behavior linked to religious beliefs?

There is no future in staying the same

There is a tendency in many of us to resist change. We're all creatures of habit, embracing the familiar, and finding comfort in customary routines. Unfortunately, the less adaptable we are to inner (personal) and outer (worldly) changes in our environment, the more vulnerable we become.

Darwin wrote: "It is not the most intelligent of the species that survives, it is not the strongest that survives, the species that survives is the one best able to adapt and adjust to the changing environment that one finds themselves in." I'll add that change isn't limited to our external environment, but also adjusting to our strengths and weaknesses; and the different stages of life, from growth to coping with old age.

Acting in our own best interest requires that we have good self-awareness and self-appraisal to meet the challenges of our ever-changing personal circumstances. Denial fueled by emotion is the irrational and self-destructive attempt to stay the same, and hope the problem goes away. When the boat is sinking, you can't keep doing things the same old way. The problem then is not the problem—the problem is the failure to adjust to changing circumstances.

The pages that follow will elaborate and expand upon the five principles. I will relate the histories of a number of my patients (disguised of course) and public figures to bring these principles to life. My ultimate goal is to provide information that will enable people to live better. The near term goals are as follows:

- Answer the questions posed
- Bring to life the five principles
- Go beyond understanding to execution

PART ONE

Acting in Your Own Best Interest

(AIYOBI)

Acting in Your Own Best Interest

The best advice you can give anyone is to Act In Your Own Best Interest. That seems simple enough, doesn't it, but don't confuse self-interest with selfish behavior. Self-interest refers to behavior that promotes well-being and enables us to not only survive but thrive. The way we conduct our lives is an essential barometer of our mental health.

How would you define mental health or, for that matter, mental illness? What comes to mind? Neither are easy questions to answer. A standard dictionary definition of mental illness is: "any disease of the mind." Mental health is often defined as "a person's condition with regard to their psychological and emotional well being." That sounds like a lot of double talk to me, remarkably lacking in descriptive clarity. I suggest another perspective, a definition that is clear, timely, and empowering:

Acting in your own best interest (AIYOBI) is good mental health!

A reasonably healthy person tends to avoid activities that ultimately result in pain, loss, and death. What better defines mental illness than engaging in behavior that is harmful to oneself? This holds true, regardless of one's symptoms or diagnosis. Self-destructive behavior profoundly sabotages our well-being. We are all mentally ill to the extent that we engage in behavior that is not in our best interest.

A Measure of Mental Health

If we consider whether we act in our own best interest as a measure of mental health, it unveils a new perspective that has definite advantages. First, it is current, we do not depend on some historical diagnosis, but instead, examine the here and now of our behavior. Secondly, it is specific. You can have a diagnosis of schizophrenia, yet engage in healthy, beneficial behavior. Or, you can be a highly successful physician who is under burdensome debt because of his Las Vegas gambling. In that area of his life, he is undoubtedly mentally ill.

Further, the measure is empowering. We are not merely the victims of the disorder, but we have control. Our mental health is in our own hands, depending on the choices we make. Using the *AIYOBI* principle as a measure makes it easier to talk about any potential problems with a true friend. Asking, "Do you think this would be in my best interest?" is preferable to talking about symptoms. The measure is forward-looking and functionally relevant. A label doesn't help anybody.

* * *

There is much in life that is beyond our control. At times, we are all victims of unfair treatment and painful misfortune, but where we do have control, we often squander it with self-destructive behavior. Self-injurious behavior often transcends all aspects of living, most notably, our relationships, our work, our health, and our self-esteem. What is it then, that drives us to sabotage ourselves? It's not a mystery. The perennial causes of our self-inflicted wounds are our emotions. As I said before you can be a genius and self-destructive. Our emotions have a very low IQ.

What is it about emotions that drive us to make the same stupid mistakes over and over again? We know emotions have enormous power because when we are in the grip of one, whether it be fear, love, jealousy, or rage, the emotion ultimately takes over, making it difficult to think clearly. Emotionally charged thoughts conquer reason, and we behave in ways that are difficult to control. Unfortunately, when emotions are at the helm and directing our behavior, we are at the precipice of disaster.

Sometimes we can foresee the error of our ways before we act, but reason and logic can be weak competitors for the raw power of emotion. Ask O. J. Simpson (jealous rage), President Clinton (lust), Bernard Madoff (greed), whether or not they knew better. Although O. J. Simpson was found not guilty of killing his ex-wife, most clear-minded people believe he was guilty. The fact that he had a history of domestic violence made it an easy crime to solve.

We'd have to ask who is in charge, lust, or reason if you trust a 19-year-old intern for oral sex in the White House? What about the multimillionaire who risks everything to steal his clients' money in a massive Ponzi scheme?

We're talking about three successful, intelligent men that self-destructed even though they knew better. It's not like they didn't understand the risks; they didn't care. Their urges and sense of entitlement ruled their behavior. I am never surprised when a sociopath hurts others. But it is their failure to recognize their imminent demise in the very action they are taking, which is astonishing.

We can all look back at times where we have sabotaged

ourselves. We know better, but we surrender to the compulsion or intense feeling that grips us. Emotion has no intellect. There is no logic to our lustful urges or our irrational worries. They reside in the primitive part of our brain that lacks judgment. Everyone's emotions are primitive, and our emotions are no more irrational than those of the Supreme Court Justices. When emotion overpowers good sense resulting in self-harm, we are essentially turning against ourselves and, therefore, mentally ill. Not always in the clinical sense, but in the bigger picture, self-injurious behavior is pathological.

Our Appetites

Too often, our unhealthy appetites undermine our well being. The obvious examples include food—sadly, the worldwide obesity rate has nearly tripled since 1975—sex, alcohol, and drugs. Each of these appetites leaves us profoundly vulnerable to our emotional yearnings. We overeat to obesity and serious illness. We take pills for diabetes because it's easier than curbing our appetite.

One day, walking on the beach, I saw a man get knocked over by a wave in waist-deep water. It was about eight in the evening, and no one else was around. The elderly man could not get up and began to panic. He was drowning in three feet of water. I went in and used all of my strength to help him to his feet. As I walked him out, he thanked me with deep appreciation. He was about a hundred pounds over-weight. I couldn't get this thought out of my head for some time, how does someone do that to themselves? To virtually disable themselves for food.

Why is it so difficult to control the type and amount of food we consume when the consequences are so dire? Is food so powerful that it controls us? No, but the feeling and emotions associated with food are in control. Food is our reward, our tranquilizer, and it's immediately gratifying. It comforts us and never rejects us. We eat to ease the pain when we are sad, lonely, and bored. And then eat some more to help us fall asleep.

As with food, we numb ourselves with excessive amounts of alcohol, opiates, and other quick-fix substances. We love the way it makes us feel. The immediacy, the feeling of lightness and pleasure as the pain fades away. When you're hurting, it feels good to be "comfortably numb." What stops most of us from taking that path are the consequences.

Addiction, whether food or drugs or other dangerous behavior, is the model for self-sabotage. While it might seem out of touch, I do not consider addiction to be a disease. There is no disease process, no invasion of organisms. We are turning against ourselves, permitting our yearnings to take control even when we know better. Yes, addiction has a genetic component. The genetically predisposed are more vulnerable to the cravings and rewards of drugs and alcohol. We all have genetic predispositions that we have to live with, both good and bad. We're dealt those cards, and we have to live with them. Our genes don't pour that extra drink or shoot drugs through our veins. We make a choice to take the fix because it feels good right now. Consequences be damned. When feelings and emotions are in control, there is no limit to our excess and the eventual toxic outcome.

Alcohol and drugs have the capacity to make most of us feel good. They're fast-acting, pleasurable, and require little effort. When reason and logic are in control, we know when to stop. We recognize the danger and never give any substance control over our life. We understand the profound consequences of escaping into a life of intoxication. Most of us have seen a family member, a friend, or a neighbor take the painful spiral down from Wall Street and cashmere to rags and the gutter.

The Addiction of Excess

It is not just addictions to food, alcohol, and drugs that cause harm, but so too the addiction of excess. Richard and I became acquainted while working at the same hospital. There was nothing that Richard wanted that he didn't acquire. He was a highly successful anesthesiologist with an income of about a half a million a year. Unfortunately, his appetite demanded more.

He drove his Porsche to his plane from his home in the city to his place at the sea. He was *so vain* that he went to Saratoga and bought thoroughbreds on borrowed money. "I'm going to win the Kentucky Derby," he once told me. But it all ended badly for Richard: bankruptcy, a tax fraud conviction, and divorce. When the size of our home, the brand of our car, and the designer of our clothes define us, we're on shaky ground.

Our Relationships

Our feelings can lead us down a dark path in our relationships. We may be blindly attracted to the wrong people because they have a certain charisma that seduces us. We may see signs of questionable moral behavior but look the other way. We fool ourselves because of our need for acceptance. Our desperation to be liked makes us vulnerable and hurts us in the end. Fifty women or more could not resist the good looks and superficial charm of Ted Bundy. He was so devious that for a time, he worked as a telephone counselor at the Seattle Crisis Clinic.

Spending time with people who make us feel good about ourselves seems like the right thing to do. After all, why would we pursue people who mistreat us? Perhaps, the answer lies in the Groucho Marx joke: "I would never join a club that would accept me as a member." When we have low self-esteem, we tend to see others who are attracted to us as losers. As a result, we pursue those individuals we view as *better* than us in the hope of elevating our worth. Very often, we are chasing after the enemy.

Carla, a six-foot-tall Latina beauty, attracted the most popular boys in high school. They all made runs at her, but to Carla, they were boys, too immature and way too boring. After high school, Carla enrolled at the nearby community college and took a part-time job at Starbucks.

John, one of her regular customers, caught her eye. He was 26, seven years older, handsome, funny, and totally cool. When John came through the door of the coffee shop, she could feel her pulse quicken. Before long, they had their first date, and John showed up in the most beautiful silver sports car she'd ever seen. That night they went to an exclusive restaurant where they drank martinis and two bottles of red wine. They ate food that Carla never knew existed. Flushed by the wine, feeling high and excited, Carla knew she had finally found someone special.

John was on the phone when the bill came, and Carla gasped at the amount. Everything they had eaten and drank came to more than $400. John paid the bill with five $100 bills, and for a moment, Carla wondered if he was involved in something illegal. Back at his apartment that evening, John was gentle and self-confident, unlike the nervous little boys in high school.

Carla became his regular girl, and after only a few weeks, he asked her to move in. Carla couldn't say yes fast enough. His apartment was on the 27th floor with great views of the river. She thought how lucky she was—*He has it all: he's rich, good looking, smart, and best of all, he's mine.*

A few months down the road, the shine wore off. John exhibited a dark side that at times frightened her. He often lost his temper with people on the phone, and she came in for her share of grief, as well. One day he exploded at her because the music was too loud. John told Carla he had a distribution job and worked crazy late-night hours because he had to arrange all the logistics for morning deliveries. Carla was quick to forgive his occasional loss of temper; no one is perfect, she thought. Carla's heart trumped all reasonable thoughts of concern.

I first met Carla in the brain injury unit of the hospital where I worked. Her chart said she was 19, but it was hard to tell. A bullet had entered the back of her head behind her right ear and exited through her eye socket. I learned this was the result of a drug deal gone bad. She had been in the passenger seat when she caught a bullet meant for John.

Carla's life was over, but John escaped unscathed. He visited her once in the hospital and then disappeared. Carla chased the enemy, caught him, and then lost everything.

Another case of chasing the enemy goes back to my early days while working at Manhattan State Psychiatric Hospital. Barbara and I were colleagues of a sort, but we never met since we worked on different floors. I couldn't even tell you what she looked like, but both of us were psychologists working at Manhattan State.

The hospital sometimes admitted psychiatric patients that had committed crimes but required treatment for serious mental illness. Jim had murdered his wife and was found guilty. After being diagnosed with schizophrenia, the court sent him to our hospital and admitted him to Barbara's unit. They told me Jim was an engaging guy. He had the staff laughing at his jokes, and at times they even forgot he was a murderer.

Jim had brazen charm and charisma and seduced Barbara. All her training went out the window when irrational emotion prevailed over reason. Her strong attraction to Jim sabotaged her clinical judgment. Foolishly, she thought she was in control. Barbara wrote him weekend passes, which were prohibited due to his murder conviction. She not only wrote him passes but brought him home to spend weekends with her. This story doesn't have a happy ending, as you can imagine. They found Barbara murdered in her bed. Jim escaped and was never found. Many years later, I saw the story depicted on *America's Most Wanted*.

* * *

Is there anything more destructive than jealousy? Jealous behavior produces the exact opposite of our intent. A former patient of mine had become convinced her husband was having an affair. She began calling him at work multiple times a day, something she had never done before. She would show up unexpectedly at his office to check on him, offering some ridiculous excuse for being there. Even when her husband was home with her, she couldn't contain her jealous angst. She conducted an inquisition on the poor man, bombarding him with questions. Why are you so late? Where did you go? Who did you see? What time will you be home tomorrow? Whining, "You have time for everybody but me."

Instead of drawing him closer, her behavior had the opposite reaction. She was driving him away. If she had intended to make herself as unattractive as possible, she succeeded.

The more we pursue someone, trying to make them ours, the faster they run in the opposite direction. If there were a law of relationship physics, it would state, the more needy and dependent we are, the more unappealing we become. Logically, many of us understand this dynamic but find it hard to control. We know that self-reliance and being more independent is the answer, but our neediness subverts us.

Dependency is the leading cause of chronic bad treatment. Otherwise, you just walk out the door. Women who remain in abusive relationships are engaging in self-sabotage. They live in denial, fueled by fear of being alone, dependency, and feelings of inadequacy. Their hope is it will be different next time. It never is. The best predictor of future violence is past violent behavior.

Our Work

Work provides us with many ways to shoot ourselves in the foot. Recently, we've seen an avalanche of predatory sexual conduct cases come to light in the fields of entertainment, politics, the media, and business. Stealing from the company and coming to work under the influence are also sure-fire ways to sabotage one's career. Those being extreme cases, for most of us, two fundamental factors determine whether or not we find success on the job.

First, I ask if the person is in the right position? Do we know our attributes, our strengths, and our weaknesses? We do ourselves an injustice when we enter a line of work for which we're not suited. A sales job is probably not the best career path if you're an introvert. Knowing ourselves as it relates to work depends upon accurate self-appraisal. Our uniqueness, what we are really good at, will serve us well when we find the right vehicle, no matter the job, an auto mechanic, social worker, salesman, or scientist.

Secondly, but most importantly, be the best you can be. We sabotage ourselves at work when we deliver a mediocre performance, doing just enough to get by. Whether this lack of effort is due to resentment, laziness, boredom, or ignorance, a poor performance takes us down the path of self-inflicted pain. You have power because of your expertise. When you know your job better than anyone else, you have independence. When you're the best at your job, you're not trapped. You need not be a victim of bad bosses and lousy working conditions. Interestingly, these are the most common complaints, not the work itself.

In most cases, when we are really good at what we do, we will be appreciated and valued, and that makes work so much sweeter. If we feel unappreciated or overlooked, knowing we have the "goods," we can take our talent anywhere. Hard work pays off, giving us our liberty and respect.

The most important determinant of success is not intelligence, but the drive and persistence to be the best you can be. I've seen this play out over and over again. Average intelligence is sufficient to succeed at most any endeavor. It is the dedication to hard work and perseverance that defines our future.

We are not limited by our intellect, but by our willingness to strive for excellence.

A Tale of Two Cases

Steve, 24, attended a good university, worked hard, and graduated with an above-average GPA. His major was economics, and he got a job on Wall Street right out of college. The economy was booming, and jobs were plentiful. By the time I saw Steve, he had been let go from five firms in the course of two years. He had no problem getting hired but barely made it past a few months before being terminated.

In our first session, I recognized evidence of his immaturity, and problems with self-awareness and social judgment, which suggested executive function problems. Further interviews and neuropsychological testing revealed deficits in frontal lobe functioning. The issues were not related to intelligence or knowledge, but rather social skills, volition, and the flexibility necessary for adapting to the fast-paced environment of Wall Street.

Talking with his mother, I learned of a birth complication in which he may have suffered oxygen deprivation for an unknown period. This complication was all forgotten as Steve excelled as a student right through college. Executive function deficits often go undetected in the academic environment, but surface in jobs in which initiative, social judgment, planning, and adapting are sorely tested.

It was apparent to me that Steve's future was not on Wall Street but in a job with more structure and less pressure. Steve was open, honest, and appreciated our sessions together. He was a great young man, and I thoroughly enjoyed working with him. My guidance to Steve was that he would fare much better in a more structured environment where his skills could flourish. Steve liked math and enjoyed keeping all kinds of statistical probabilities on his favorite baseball, football, and basketball teams. Those were his strengths, and we talked about the types of jobs where he could employ his abilities.

Soon after our talks, Steve applied for a position with a large insurance company. Steve had found something that matched his talents, and he thrived in the new job. The last time I heard from him, he had been working as an actuarial agent with the same company for eleven years.

* * *

Mark, 44, reluctantly came to see me, pressured by his wife's constant nagging, as he put it. Mark was a sales manager in the tech industry and had moved cross-country four times to new jobs in the last three years before he became my patient. This upheaval affected not only Mark and his wife Carolyn but also their three school-aged children.

Mark had been either fired or quit each job. Of course, he had a different boss story for each of those lost jobs. There was the story of a horrible boss who knew nothing. And a tale of the supervisor who was out to get him because he felt threatened that Mark knew so much more than he did. Another nervous boss watched him like a hawk and criticized his every move. Then, there was the obnoxious boss who made Mark chauffeur him around, drink with him, and listen to his boring stories. On his last job, the working conditions were so bad he said it was like working in a sweatshop.

Not once did Mark take any responsibility for his string of defeats. It was never his fault. It was always about how stupid and incompetent someone else was. One day after a number of sessions, I said to him, "Maybe the problem is you, Mark. Either it's your attitude, or maybe you're not as good as you think you are."

Mark's head seemed to swell, his face reddened, his eyes bulged, and he told me I was stupid, that I had no idea what I was talking about. "This is a waste of my time," he bellowed, walking toward the door. "I'm never coming back."

And he didn't.

Perhaps, I could have done a better job and established a better relationship with Mark, but he was closed and rigid.

To him, I was just another one of his bosses.

Feelings and Emotions

While feelings and emotions are the culprits for much of our self-inflicted misery, they are also the power source for our excitement, joy, and love. Emotions are the "Air Beneath Our Wings," they are life's energy source. Without these emotions, existence would be very boring. They can be a great source of pleasure, but at times may lead us down a path of self-annihilation. It all depends on our judgment and self-control.

At this juncture, it would be helpful to define what we generally mean by feelings and emotions. A feeling is a general state of being. For example, I feel blue, anxious, tired, or bored are all examples of states of being. Our emotions are more targeted and specific. So, we fear something specific, like sharks, or we love our dog. Our anger and rage are also more typically targeted. If we're wading in the ocean and see a shark swimming towards us, that produces fear and propels us to swim like crazy. On the other hand, when we swim in the ocean and worry something terrible might happen, that's anxiety.

Fear is an emotion that is central to our survival. Good

fortune is finding ourselves wired with just the right amount of fear. Too little fear and we run the risk of self-destruction. When we're not sufficiently risk aversive, we engage in irrational behavior that will eventually lead to our harm or demise. The road to financial independence does not run through Las Vegas.

Too much fear may cause us to live a life of psychic pain and paralysis. We spend our days thinking something bad is always about to happen, that there's danger everywhere. Why get in the car and go somewhere when we may get into an accident? Visit New York? Never! The hotels are infested with bedbugs, and tuberculosis is once again on the rise. Can you see that fear is a thief, and its victims are pleasure and peace of mind?

Fear is irrational when it is inappropriate for a particular individual and situation. Who then is to decide what is too much or too little fear? It cannot be the emotion fear itself because emotion is not logical or rational. Reason must prevail. I would love to climb Mt. Everest, but I know I'm not prepared. Even if you are fearless, a risk-taker, good judgment must be your pilot. It's not wise to fly your plane over the ocean at night without instrument training. It is not reasonable to have sex in the White House even though your fear of getting caught is not palpable.

Fear and all other emotions are our brain's more primitive expression of being human. Our feelings and yearnings are difficult to control. We are often told we can change the way we feel. "Why do you feel that way?" they ask us. How we feel is hard to change by just trying to do so. It's like trying to drive a car with the engine turned off. Action is the source of change. When you act in your own best interest, you will ultimately feel better.

When you're feeling anxious, depressed, completely down on yourself, it's hard to reason. Anxiety is relentless. It finds threats everywhere and takes control. You may pace around the room, trying to think more positively, but it feels impossible. Anxiety has a strong physiological component. In the grip of anxiety, you find yourself sweating, trying to catch your breath, and your heart is racing. These physical symptoms supercharge fearful thoughts.

If we can alleviate or at least reduce the impact of the physical symptoms, we can think more clearly. Running, swimming, or vigorous exercise of any kind are great ways to burn off the angst. Meditation, long walks on the beach, and medication such as Xanax can help diffuse the nasty physical symptoms. Once we take a deep breath and gather ourselves, we begin to feel better and think more rationally.

Depression's dark thoughts have their own neurobiological components, fueling feelings of dread. Depleted, it feels like we're walking underwater; every step is an effort. People suffering from depression are caught in a never-ending nightmare affecting body and mind. They're burdened with feelings of failure, loneliness, and fears of terrible things to come weigh heavily on them. You may not want to get out of bed, but fighting depression requires taking action in your best interest. It helps to have an ally (a spouse, friend, or therapist) facilitate Engagement, Exercise, Medication, and Therapy. Once we loosen the grip of despair that dominates our being, we can begin to think more rationally.

Quite different from a biologically based depression is normal depression. Normal depression is when we feel sad in response to loss and disappointment. When we lose a loved one or suffer through a divorce, should we not feel sad? To that point, we are way over medicated. Pharmaceutical advertising, plastered everywhere in all forms of media, certainly plays a role. It seems like half the population is on antidepressants. They may have little beneficial effect, but once started, we're too afraid to stop.

* * *

Most of the time, knowing what is in our own best interest is quite apparent. We know when we overeat, drink too much, and sabotage our relationships, yet we do it anyway. We can't resist pleasurable foods even though shortly after we've finished eating, we feel miserable. We find our attractive neighbor irresistible even though we know it will lead to disaster.

When emotions steer one's life decisions, we behave like a rudderless ship in a turbulent sea. Recently, we have all been witness to how compulsive lust has led to pain and suffering for not only the victims but the perpetrators as well. Harvey Weinstein, Bill Cosby, and Anthony Weiner are examples of some of the most powerful people in our country who self-destructed when falling prey to irrational urges. While you can argue that they deserve to suffer, it is the self-annihilation and the dreadful shame they bring upon themselves that is shocking. It enlightens us to the power and blindness of their primitive yearnings.

Reason Over Emotion

Who's in the driver's seat? Do feelings and emotions drive our actions even though we know better? "I love that meatball parmesan hero. So, what if it's fattening and gives me heartburn. It's worth it!" Clearly, feelings are the winner here. It is truly amazing that for the very short-term pleasures of food, we wreck our goals of feeling healthy and fit and looking good.

What is it about food that has such power over us? Nothing! It is not the food but the perceived pleasure that it brings. That yearning …

"I know I shouldn't call him. I just can't help myself." Clearly, emotion is in control here as well. Jealousy represents a clear and compelling illustration of how self-destructive behavior driven by emotions can be. The more possessive we become, the more we display our neediness and dependency, the more unattractive we become. When we are jealous, we act irrationally. We sabotage the relationship that we hold so dearly. "Where were you? Who were you with? You have time for everybody but me." The very goal of holding on to the person is subverted by uncontrollable needy behavior. One may know that we'd fare better by being a bit elusive and independent, but it is difficult to control.

How many times have we said, "I don't feel like doing it." That negative feeling may refer to going to work, studying for a test, paying taxes, or cleaning the house. The truth is what we feel like doing has nothing to do with reality. We often sabotage our success because "we don't feel like it." When we understand that life is a working proposition, we accept that what we feel like doing has nothing to do with the demands of reality.

Achievement and success are incredibly gratifying. They are built on the foundation of hard work and discipline. Nothing worthwhile was ever created by a person who "didn't feel like doing it." We harm ourselves when we fall prey to the childhood emotion of only wanting to do what we feel like doing. Reasonable and mature adults clearly understand that life demands much more than what we feel like doing. Except for our pets, most animals who only do what they feel like doing don't survive very long.

The key to achievement is the ability to delay gratification. Our feelings and emotions demand immediate results, instant pleasure. Emotions demonstrate no ability to delay gratification. Food gives us immediate pleasure. Not doing an arduous task brings us relief. Feelings are not long-term propositions; they drive us to seek quick resolutions. In contrast, success in life demands discipline and the desire to work toward future goals. Metaphorically, we need to give up the short-term blissful pleasure of pizza for the much more rewarding achievement of being healthy, physically fit, and looking attractive.

Lifetime achievement may be inspired by emotion, but it's accomplished by the employment of reason. Establishing a powerful, rational inner voice is essential for living well. In our relationships, work, finances, and self-appraisal, reason must prevail over feelings. Think of it as an inner dialogue between the rational you and the irrational you. When the rational you wins out, success is at hand. The rational you says one or two glasses of wine is quite enough because you'll be driving home in the dark. The rational you says I'd better prepare for that business meeting tomorrow rather than watching Monday Night Football. The rational you says if I have a bottle of water instead of that ice cream sundae, I'll feel much better an hour from now. The rational you says don't chase after her because the harder you pursue, the faster she'll run.

Are there times in life when what is in our best interest is not apparent? Of course. We all have to make complicated decisions involving career, health, and finance, where there may be little clarity. In these situations, reason doesn't have a solid footing. We can study the issues and develop some expertise, but to succeed and live well, we need accurate self-appraisal.

Accurate Self-Appraisal

Generally, we know what is in our best interest. There are times, however, when we are stumbling in the dark. When we don't know the right choice to make, is it the task at hand that we don't understand, or is it ourselves? Self-knowledge is an essential component of *AIYOBI*. It enables us to make the right decision in complex situations.

Deciding on the best course of treatment for a serious illness requires research. Choosing the right college or the best company to work for takes research. But that is only half the equation, how do you research yourself? How can you know what is in your best interest if you genuinely don't know yourself? While most of us think we pretty much know who we are, denial is our treacherous enemy. We have all seen denial at work. Most obvious is the alcoholic, whose excessive drinking is eroding his or her work and family life and, when confronted, refuses to acknowledge reality. Mental illness and reality are not highly correlated.

While denial may not be a fully conscious process, its intent is clear. It is to avoid reality. We employ denial when we fail to seek medical attention for symptoms that we explain away with magical thinking. We use denial when we are in lust with someone and look the other way when his or her dark side emerges. When things fall apart, and we always find someone else to blame, we're usually in denial. Denial is the failure to accept the truth. It occurs when our fear or greed or rage, overpowers good judgment. Unfortunately, denial, the rejection of reality, almost always leads to bad outcomes. Ironically, we can often recognize denial in others, but not in ourselves.

AIYOBI requires dedication to the truth. So, how do we research ourselves and discover our truth? Such research may require an honest look at our personal history through introspection, intimate discussions with people we trust, and therapy. These are all paths leading to self-enlightenment. Ideally, therapy is an educational process in which the therapist's goal is to understand the patient, win over their trust, and then guide them to *AIYOBI*. A good therapist can be a great ally in fostering self-awareness and facilitating growth.

Irrational Me vs. Rational Me

Is it possible to be your own therapist? It is a difficult task, but to the degree we can have an honest inner dialogue, we can achieve beneficial results. Thoughtful reflection and dedication to the truth are crucial elements. The goal, whatever the issue or conflict, should be to differentiate the rational from the irrational. The irrational is always going to be how we feel. Our rational voice tells us what is logical and moral. Our rational voice examines our feelings, urges, and emotions in the light of reality and what is in our best interest. For example:

I wake up worried that I have the flu. I'm nervous and feel like I have a fever and take my temperature. It's 97.6. Reason tells me I'm okay, relax, let go of the fear.

On my drive to work, some jerk cuts me off and makes me slam on the brakes. My rage boils to the surface. My voice of reason says stay calm, don't be a jerk like him, or you will be fighting battles every day.

Let's consider some of the characters we discussed previously. For Bill Clinton, the lustful fantasy appeared before him as a nineteen-year-old intern. His yearning demanded immediate gratification. Now, let's be Bill Clinton's rational voice, "Do I trust this nineteen-year-old girl that I hardly know? Will she keep it a secret or tell the world? Are the risks too great here? Are a few minutes of pleasure worth the potential pain?" If Bill had this inner dialogue and paid attention to his rational voice, the answer would have been NO, it's not worth it.

Let us try and get into the head of O. J. Simpson. He was clearly enraged by being rejected by his ex-wife, Nicole Simpson. His sense of entitlement and jealous rage propelled him to murder his wife and her friend Ron Goldman. Let's become the rational voice inside O. J.'s head. "If you do this, you will not only destroy her but destroy yourself. As her ex-husband, you will be the number one suspect. There is no way your alibi is going to work. There are so many beautiful women available to you. Take some time to let your fury pass. Don't destroy both her and yourself." Clearly, O. J.'s rational voice was either absent or lost out to his rage.

These two dramatic cases of famous people are purely for illustration. We've all had our own experiences, where our rational side lost to our irrational yearning. Maybe it was a bad financial investment prompted by greed. Bernie Madoff swindled many extremely intelligent and wealthy people. Had they employed their rational voice, they could've overcome their greed. Their rational voice should have told them there is no one who can guarantee a 12% return in up and down markets. Greed is not good. It's stupid because emotion has a very low IQ.

If we take the time to listen to our rational voice daily, we can make beneficial strides in *AIYOBI*. Whatever the dilemma or decision might be, identify what the feelings, emotions, and yearnings are, and then evaluate them in the light of reason before taking action. Ask yourself:

- Is this really in my best interest?
- Why am I doing this, and what are the possible consequences?
- Who is in control? Good judgment or fantasy, primitive wishful thinking?
- What is the Risk vs. Reward equation look like? Am I taking on too much risk for a small gain?

No matter what the issue may be—investments, medical decisions, relationships, career decisions—ask if the potential benefits outweigh the downside.

* * *

Irrational fear and worry are debilitating villains, and they punish day after day. When fear is our enemy, a calming rational voice can counter the concern. Self-talk such as: "*Instead of anticipating the very worst, wait till it happens and then deal with it!" "Worry is forever and accomplishes noth-ing." "Fear, I'm not going to listen to you or give you any cred-ibility, you've cost me dearly, and you're always wrong."*

Humor is an excellent tonic in these cases. Sometimes we can laugh at our troubles and ourselves. Talk to a true friend to get an objective view. Revealing oneself to intimate others is often therapeutic and strengthens the relation-ship. Think of your history and all the times you worried for nothing. As discussed previously, anxiety has a strong physiological component, so consider exercise, meditation, music, or a glass of wine to help defuse the angst. Use your inner dialogue to learn from the experience and mistakes of others. Mathematical probability is a great reality check for some of the most common fears. The odds of being struck by lightning in our lifetime are one in 15,000. How about being killed by a shark? The odds of that happening are one in 3,000,000.

When we pay attention to our rational voice, we can more clearly see which path to take. We can recognize when our primitive brain (emotion) is taking us off track. How-ever, knowing is not enough. Establishing a powerful ratio-nal voice is essential, but not sufficient. The hardest part is the execution.

Execution

Knowing what is in our best interest has its hurdles, but it is far easier than changing our behavior. Execution, particularly early in the process of facing a challenge, is demanding and requires extraordinary effort and discipline. Execution is fueled by desire, forged by delay of gratification, and dependent on resiliency for the times we slip up.

We are unlikely to exert the effort if we don't like and respect ourselves. When we love someone, we aim to act in his or her best interest. We try to foster their growth, a healthy lifestyle, and good self-esteem. If we can act in such a positive fashion for someone else, why not for ourselves? Not loving ourselves is irrational. It is a twisted feeling that is in opposition to the laws of nature and self-preservation.

How we feel about ourselves is an acid test of the inner dialogue between the irrational Me and the rational Me. Self-loathing is irrational, it is the bricks and mortar of pain and suffering. If you find it hard to like your present self, then engage in good deeds that will enhance your self-esteem, enter therapy and only spend time with people that treat you with respect.

When we successfully execute, we bridge the gap between knowledge and action. In therapy, a major goal is to educate patients about themselves. Increasing self-awareness is the easy part. It is the changing of behavior that is most daunting. "I know," and "I just can't control myself," are typical replies to questions about our failure to execute self-control.

Where does the power for self-control reside? Not surprisingly, it's in the brain, and for the most part, in the frontal lobe. Self-control is dependent upon what neuroscientists call our executive functions. Our executive functions are the engine for self-regulation. They involve volition, the capacity for goal-oriented behavior, planning, and effective performance. It is the job of the frontal lobes, the more advanced part of our brain, to control and regulate urges of the more primitive part of the brain. There are many syndromes where neurological impairment leads to poor self-regulation, such as trauma, hypoxia, and ADHD. In such instances, neuropsychological therapy works toward improving one's competence for self-regulation.

Similarly, civilization depends on laws, which demand self-control. We are not permitted to steal our neighbor's wife and car simply because we are stronger than the neighbor. Society establishes rules to hold in check irrational and predatory behavior on the part of its citizens. Returning to the word executive (execute), it is the responsibility of the executive branch of government to enforce self-control of its constituents. Taking an historical view, similar to us as individuals there are many governments that are not up to the task. Governments led by frenzied irrational emotion gave us Adolph Hitler, Nazi Germany, and WW ll.

What then is the key for turning the rational into action? First must come the desire to change. Without the motivation to change there will be no change. Sociopaths (anti-social personality) are typically not suffering this angst because they have no desire to change, and therapy is a waste of time with them. Whether we are disgusted with ourselves, tired of suffering, or whatever, if the drive to change is absent, we will continue along the path of self-harm.

Successful execution requires the ability to delay gratification. Can you surrender the immediate pleasure of eating donuts every day to feel better about yourself a month or two down the road? Will you study for your final exams over the weekend or drink yourself into oblivion? Can you control your jealous whining? Are you strong enough to make that sacrifice and give up your need for immediate gratification?

Generally, we can say that the easy road is usually the most troublesome path for us.

Success hinges on the willingness to do the work of the executive branch. Who is in charge, our primitive brain where emotion resides, or the more advanced part of our brain that knows better? Each of us is the executive in charge, and as it relates to our own lives, we have the power of the Presidency.

HABIT is the best way to overcome resistance to change. As we force ourselves to engage in the desired behavior daily, resistance weakens. The HABIT gives us time to reap the rewards of our new behavior. Trusting the HABIT takes on a momentum of its own. The sacrifice we make for future gain becomes much less painful as time moves forward. Eventually, it is not a sacrifice but a more joyful way of living. We no longer miss the pizza and truly enjoy a fresh bowl of fruit.

Finally, to successfully execute, we need resiliency—the ability to get up off the canvas when we fall. There are times we regress, weaken, and fail. Backsliding is all part of the process of growth. One day's failure shouldn't shake your persistence. Sure, I ate the whole pizza, but I'll return to my sensible diet and eat healthier tomorrow. All is not lost.

I use food, both literally and figuratively, because it is profoundly illustrative of the challenge of self-control and delay of gratification. *AIYOBI* AND YOU WILL FEEL BETTER!

PART TWO

Why Be Moral

What is Moral is in Our Best Interest

Do you think you're moral? Most people think they are. We all like to believe we're moral, but what does being moral mean? When we say that someone is intelligent, it is clear what the trait describes. We don't share that common ground as it relates to moral values.

How do we evaluate the moral character of our friends? Is it their charity, views on social issues, what they tell us about themselves, or how they treat us? Other than the most obvious situations, do we recognize when we are behaving immorally? What do we consider to be immoral behavior in people we know? While our moral conduct defines our character, our ability to discern moral integrity in others may determine our fate.

Many years ago, I was asked to join a discussion group. Most of the time, we sat around drinking wine and talked seriously about little of significance. One afternoon, the discussion turned to the issue of morality. An attorney, who looked to be about 50, spoke with passion and conviction, saying, "It is my religious faith and my belief in God that gives me morality. Absent my religious beliefs, what would stop me from killing my neighbor and taking whatever I desired from him?"

A physician in the group agreed, adding, "Everything I have learned about morality came from my religious studies. I believe if you exclude religion, morality is beyond man's reach."

I objected to the notion that morality was dependent on religious faith. I argued that the same human brain, capable of solving complex problems, creating art and music, and amazing technological advances, has the capacity to develop highly reasoned moral standards.

We were a mixed group talking about declining social values, sex and violence, and our immoral political leaders. What was clear was that there was little consensus on defining what morality is. Making the issue even more confusing, our culture often elevates style over substance, technology over content, and engages in celebrity worship. I thought to myself we need a better understanding, a framework, standards of conduct that most of us can agree upon.

Lawrence Kohlberg, a Harvard Professor and founder of

The Center For Moral Education, accomplished this some 50 years ago. A student of Piaget, Kohlberg, believed individuals progressed in their moral reasoning through a series of stages similar to cognitive development.

Kohlberg was passionate about the study of morality. He was a brilliant innovator in a field virtually ignored by traditional psychology. He developed a qualitative analysis of moral conduct, which is both timeless and universal. Kohlberg traveled extensively researching moral development in diverse cultures across the world. His mission to bring moral development to light was cut short by his own hand. In January of 1987, Kohlberg, age 59, and at the apex of his career, walked into the icy waters of Boston Harbor. He was reportedly in chronic pain as the result of a parasitic infection contracted in Belize. Kohlberg also had a history of depression. We sometimes try to understand a person's suicide in terms of the last thing that happened. Suicide is much more complicated than that, being influenced by a lifetime of experience and one's genetic makeup, and not simply the last incident.

Kohlberg's view of moral development is enlightening and instructive. It uncovers the qualitative differences in moral reasoning and behavior. There are three basic levels of moral conduct: Level one, **Might Makes Right**. Kohlberg's pre-Conventional stage is the most primitive; it's where power prevails. The psychopath, the schoolyard bully, dictators, and Mafia Kingpins reside here. Dominance is the key. There is no concern with right or wrong when might makes right. The most powerful people act as they wish and take what they want.

At the **Conventional Level**, our moral reasoning and behavior are in accord with society's accepted values: the rule of law, religion, and other social institutions that guide our conduct.

Kohlberg's post-Conventional and most advanced level outlines how we conduct our lives with **Independent Ethical Principles** evolving over time. Self-interest or what's politically correct doesn't influence our actions, but rather independent judgments of what is truly just. A small minority of any population, less than 10%, attains this level. Most of us reside at the Conventional level. These qualitative differences in moral reasoning and conduct can help us analyze our thoughts and behaviors and those of significant others. When power prevails, what is "right" is what the most powerful person says is right. The dynamic is the same whether that powerful person is a parent or a mob boss. In a family, a spouse may use violence, intimidation, rewards, and punishment to control family members.

In our corporate and political venues, threats of termination, financial ruin, and character assassination are often employed to force submission. In a family, classroom, or nation, the populace doesn't "go along" because of well-reasoned explanation but rather due to the leader's perceived power to bring about pleasure or pain.

At the Conventional level, our behavior conforms with the rule of law and socially sanctioned values. Good moral behavior is what society's institutions say it is, whether it is the church or the government. A family may make many of their decisions in accord with their church affiliations; politicians vote along the lines of their party, and corporate employees act in accord with company policies and procedures. There is no certainty of justice but rather conduct that is consistent with a socially sanctioned authority.

The vast majority of any population operates at the conventional level. The individual's moral reasoning and behavior are as good as the authority that he aligns himself with. This doesn't require independent thinking but rather an awareness of the appropriate rules and regulations. Research finds that most of us are in this middle ground. Interestingly, most people will tell you that they are at level three, demonstrating independent ethical principles. It feels good to believe you're supremely moral.

At the most advanced level, decisions are made based on independent judgments of what is the most ethical behavior regarding a specific situation. Morally elite individuals act on their own set of beliefs independent of power and convention, instead relying on well-reasoned ethics. The courageous morally elite are often ahead of their time, scorned they sacrifice the safety of standing with the herd. Those individuals, who violated their government's orders and hid Jews in their homes at considerable risk to themselves during the Nazi reign of terror, fit this profile.

Often, we need a historical perspective to appreciate a moral act that is ahead of the social mores of the times. Abraham Lincoln's conduct in office over a century ago is much more valued today than it was when the nation's future looked bleak during the Civil War. Slavery was a clear example of the **Might Makes Right** level of morality where one class of people through the exercise of power exploited and damaged their victims for self-gain.

Henry David Thoreau, the author of *Walden*, was born in 1817 in Concord, Massachusetts. A Harvard graduate, Thoreau was a life long fierce critic of slavery. In 1846, Thoreau refused to pay delinquent poll taxes as a protest against slavery and the Mexican-American War. He was jailed for one night and while in prison wrote the essay *On Civil Disobedience*. In the essay, Thoreau wrote of the need to prioritize one's moral conscience when in conflict with an unjust law. He emphasized the need to employ principled ethics when confronting immoral behavior on the part of authority.

In 1907, Gandhi wrote of Thoreau's profound influence on him. He praised Thoreau's moral wisdom and credited his essay as an influence on the abolition of slavery. Gandhi said of Thoreau, "He was one of the greatest and most moral men America has produced."

Thoreau's essay also influenced Martin Luther King, Jr. In his autobiography, King wrote of reading *On Civil Disobedience* several times. The essay presented him with the idea of nonviolent resistance as a means of combatting injustice. King said, "I became convinced that noncooperation with evil is as much a moral obligation as is cooperation with good. No other person has been more eloquent and passionate in getting this idea across than Henry David Thoreau. The teachings of Thoreau came alive in our civil rights movement."

Thoreau died in 1862 at the age of 44 as the result of tuberculosis. His moral courage lives on eternally.

* * *

Kohlberg designed his research to understand how people made moral decisions by examining their reasoning. In his cross-cultural research, he would present a series of moral dilemmas that he asked his subjects to solve. Here's one example:

"A child was playing with matches and accidentally set his mother's dress on fire, destroying the entire dress. Another boy was playing with a cigarette and purposely burned a small pinhole in his mother's dress. Which boy's actions were worse?"

Kohlberg was not as concerned with their answer but the reasoning process for getting there. In the above example, the concept of intent is examined.

As brilliant as Kohlberg's contribution may be, there is a problem with the research. Moral reasoning is not equivalent to moral action. We may reason at the most ethical level, but behave at the most primitive when personal desires are at hand. One's morality is defined by behavior, not thoughts or feelings, and certainly not words. Our moral behavior is tested when it affects us personally, when we're faced with pleasure-pain and gain-loss issues. While good moral reasoning is a prerequisite for good moral conduct, it is the actions we take that define our character.

The Presidency is particularly revealing of inconsistencies between moral reasoning and moral conduct. We get a clear picture of a president's public moral beliefs based on his speeches and platform. In time, we may learn much about a president's private behavior that is in conflict with his public persona. Unfortunately, too many presidents have provided us with evidence of this dual nature. Over the last sixty years, from Kennedy to Trump, there have been serious allegations of moral misconduct while in office. It's easy to espouse moral values when you're telling other people how to behave. Morality is personal. Our moral behavior is most telling when our own interests are at stake.

It may be interesting to look at the divergence between public and private acts of our political leaders, but it's much more meaningful to examine the moral integrity and conduct of the people who intimately touch our lives—our family, friends, and colleagues. In our personal universe, the significant dichotomy to examine is the gap between words and actions. Is there someone in your life operating at Level One, using power and manipulation to get what they want? Who is deserving of your trust and praise because they conduct their life with moral distinction?

If you suffer from moral anguish and find yourself examining your behavior by asking, *Did I do the right thing?* Then you are probably on the right path. Instead, we should be concerned about the person who never asks that question. Only the psychopath is free of moral anguish and doesn't benefit from the positive forces of moral pain, which can assist in the evolution of moral reasoning and the development of ethical principles.

The Development of Morality

Thomas Jefferson wrote, "All men are created equal" in The Declaration of Independence. Those familiar words were a brilliant moral goal for the birth of a new nation, but in a practical sense, nothing is further from the truth. We start on the journey of life on uneven terms, either blessed or cursed by the interaction of our genetic predispositions and our parenting. So powerful is this reality, that we may spend the rest of our lives reaping the benefits or struggling to overcome the pain and distortions.

Our Nervous System

Our nervous system and our environment shape our moral development. Let's begin by examining how our nervous system influences moral development. Our autonomic nervous system (ANS), which is outside our voluntary control, is activated by the experience of fear. When frightened, our heart begins to race, blood pressure rises, and our respiration increases. These survival mechanisms are wired into all of us, and we share them with other animals. They prepare us for fight or flight. These days we are not simply running from dangerous animals but face fear-provoking experiences in a myriad of situations. Fear is an extraordinarily powerful motivating force.

The emotion of fear is comprised of the thought or image of something we're afraid of, like dogs or an IRS audit, and the physical state the thought or image provokes. When we are terrified, we can experience a hollow feeling in our chest, difficulty breathing, and a rapid heartbeat. We sweat, our muscles tense, and we feel a pounding in our head. It is these physical reactions, controlled by the ANS, which endow the emotion of fear with power and intensity. Absent these intense physical reactions, the provoking thought or image tends to be rather benign. Whatever the situation, if we don't feel the fear in our gut, we are unlikely to alter our behavior.

Let's consider a situation where this dynamic is at work. Have you ever considered stealing something? Maybe not, but we can imagine the scenario. Picture the last time you were in a department store, walking down the aisle, checking out all the new items. Perhaps your eye is drawn to a small, expensive item that appears overpriced and could easily fit in your pocket. The thought of stealing that item would provoke fear for most of us. Fear of getting caught, being humiliated, and maybe even getting arrested. These are the thoughts and images that activate the ANS and create fear.

You pick up the item, examine the price tag as if contemplating the purchase while surreptitiously confirming no one is watching you. The more you think about slipping that tempting item into your pocket, the more your stomach churns and your heart races. The apprehension is building. So, you return the item to the shelf. Soon the intense physical reactions caused by the ANS abate, the bodily experience of fear subsides, and you immediately feel better—a physiological reward for doing the "right thing," not stealing.

It is not solely when we are about to break the law that the fear response engulfs us. Perhaps it's infidelity or a risky financial deal that causes the bodily experience of apprehension. You not only think it but feel in your gut that you did something wrong or are about to cross that line. The power of this unpleasant feeling will often result in a change in behavior to reduce stress so that we may feel mentally and physically better. So, when our thoughts alone are not sufficient to deter us from acting immorally, the bodily experience of fear supercharges the thought, and we behave morally because it makes us feel better. As Hemingway wrote, "So far about morals, I know only that what is immoral is what you feel bad after."

In time, the ANS response conditions us to avoid situations in which we feel fearful or guilty. Autonomic nervous system functioning is not uniform, however. Some individuals have an overactive ANS, while others are under active. As you would logically expect, individuals with hyper ANS tend to be more prone to fear and anxiety, while individuals with hypo ANS tend to have more shallow emotional responses because the physiological component is absent or significantly diminished. If we are biologically predisposed to elevated levels of fear, we avoid bad behavior because we anticipate the consequences. On the other end of the continuum, psychophysiological research has demonstrated a relationship between low fear [hypo ANS] and psychopathic behavior. So, if someone has an underactive ANS, does that mean they will become a psychopath? Of course not. We all can do the "right" thing regardless of our ANS if we believe in behaving honorably. One can develop thoughtful moral reasoning that leads to elite moral conduct regardless of one's ANS.

In most cases, what is essential is having loving and morally wise parents who provide an environment that instills honorable values and ethical behavior. What happens when the more primitive part of our brain doesn't scare us into doing the right thing? Our thought processes and ethics lodged in the more advanced part of our brain, the cortex, can accomplish a more cerebral result.

The experience of excessive fear as a result of a hyper ANS is harrowing and disabling. Fear is irrational and pathological when it is experienced disproportionate to actual risk. Given the enormously painful consequences of excessive fear, it is far better to attain good moral conduct as a result of ethical reasoning rather than a hyper ANS. When we learn to avoid immoral acts solely because of fear, we are functioning at a far more primitive level. The elevated morality of independent ethical principles is attained when we make decisions based on complex thought processes. Behavior that is the result of fear is consistent with a Might Makes Right morality that is absent the higher-level cognitive functions of reason, wisdom, and judgment.

Parental Influence

When we are young, our parents are Godlike—they create our world. Everything having to do with trust, love, and honor is founded in our childhood. What children see in their homes, they also assume exists in the universe. The cruel irony is many of our beliefs are shaped before we are old enough to judge right from wrong and to know what the world outside of the environment created by our parents is really like. Even in the most corrupt dictatorships, the populace has the opportunity to learn about better ways of life and then either flee or overthrow their leaders. Children have no such choice. A ten-year-old can't say to their parents, "You are too selfish and dishonest. I've had it. Goodbye."

Bad parenting, in most cases, cannot be traced back to one or more traumatic event. It is the experience of everyday living that shapes the child's view of himself and others. If a parent behaves like a bully, a cheat, and a manipulator, chances are the child will as well. Children may never fully understand the impact of toxic parenting. They tend to believe that their negative feelings about themselves and others are intrinsic to their very being.

Good parenting is cherished for life. Highly accomplished individuals in their eighties and nineties speak of their parents' love and influence as if it took place the previous day. A parent who treats others with integrity and kindness transmits this imperceptibly day by day to the very core of the child's being.

In addition to being an ethical role model, good parenting shapes the child's moral development. There are times for praise and times for admonishment, the need for corrective feedback. The best learning takes place when it is specific and immediate. We can observe how children interact with their peers. How do they relate to those who are weaker and more vulnerable, and to those stronger and seemingly invincible? A child's concern and empathy for others should be fortified, praised, tweaked, and shaped. When corrective feedback is provided with sensitivity, patience, and love, it is instructional rather than threatening or punitive. It facilitates the development of moral reasoning rather than a Might Makes Right mentality.

Punishment invoked by a parent for a child's misbehavior

is a mindless response and an erosion of legitimate authority. It teaches nothing but who holds the ultimate power: Might Makes Right. A teenage daughter comes home late from a party smelling of alcohol. The punishment is to take her phone away for a week. How is that instructive? Punishment is an easy, though morally bankrupt fix. It is the business of the Mafia and the Courts, not parents. A meaningful discussion empowers the child with wisdom rather than instilling a bully mentality.

Religion and Moral Development

What is the contribution of religion to the development of morality? A prevailing view is that a person who believes in God and knows the moral principles in the Bible is a better person for it. The sociologist, Emil Durkheim, saw religion not merely as a means of developing morality but equated religion with a moral community. He believed religion's primary purpose was to elevate man to live a more moral life than if he followed his own beliefs and desires.

The contrary argument is that faith is the antithesis of reason. What happens when the faithful fall into the hands of fanatics? A wretched leader can inspire immoral acts with a corrupt interpretation of the Bible. What if a religious leader, a perceived valid spokesman for "God," says that murder is necessary to vanquish the infidels?

Ultimately, we come back to the question of how important is religion in the development of morality. Granted that religion is used as a vehicle, a potentially powerful means for influencing moral behavior. The driver of that vehicle determines the outcome. Our parents influence most of our religious experiences. Wise parents will join a church whose teachings embrace all humanity. Toxic parents will more likely be attracted to a more perverted religious community and will use religion to provoke fear and instill hatred for those whose beliefs are different. For most of us, parental influence trumps religion. Wise and loving parents will provide a healthy moral climate regardless of their religious beliefs. Toxic parents create a treacherous moral landscape, whether they attend church or not.

Education

There is no curriculum for teaching morality in our school system. Students may learn about moral issues in their literature, history, and philosophy classes, but they are not personally relevant. Teachers and coaches may instill moral values based on their judgment, but there are no guidelines to follow. What is needed is a curriculum that looks at ethical conduct in various life circumstances.

It would not be difficult to develop an age-appropriate moral curriculum to enlighten students from first grade to college. Technology is there for our information-based searches, whether the subject is math, science, history, or language. The answers are all accessible; just turn on your tech device.

So, where do we find answers to our moral dilemmas, our conduct, and knowing the right thing to do in any situation? We face these questions every day. Is it morally wrong to copy someone else's homework? Is it morally wrong to pay someone to get your daughter into a better university? Do we really believe Grandma will fare better in assisted living, or are we tired of having to deal with her?

Solving moral problems and teaching moral reasoning requires a didactic learning experience. There is no mathematical formula. It is an experience of enlightenment. One's moral development requires thoughtful reflection, which a Google search can't provide.

The Law

The rule of law provides us with clear guidelines as to what is permissible. Most of us will abide by the rules as part of our moral conduct. Our family and our community shape our view of the legal system, the courts, the police, and the laws themselves. When we perceive the law as the enemy, the goal becomes to outwit, undermine, and prevail over it by any means possible. When the law sees the community as the enemy, injustice will occur.

Something immoral—narcissism, for example—is not illegal, and all unlawful acts like speeding are not immoral. The divergence between morality and the law is most transparent in our system of legal advocacy. Often operating at the most primitive level of morality, we find that the more money and power you have, the better your chance to influence the outcome. It would be transformative to have a legal system where both sides advocate for truth and justice.

The Hero

What is the role of the hero in enlightening and inspiring others? In life, we are sometimes fortunate enough to have a relationship or an encounter with an extraordinary person who changes us for the better. Not as the result of words or teaching, but by their actions, for the only meaningful expression of one's moral beliefs lies in action. It is through this personal relationship, with a heroic role model, that we may learn and internalize the value of sacrificing for a greater good. It may be a profound act of generosity or one of unusual courage, but it is always an act of extending oneself to aid someone less fortunate and in need of help.

Teddy P.

I was about eleven years old and standing in front of the neighborhood poolroom on Dumont Avenue when "Superman" won the day. Superman was Teddy P., a twenty-year-old, 6'3", lean but powerful basketball player. Teddy soared above the rim in the rough and tough schoolyard games of Brownsville, Brooklyn. In the 1950s, Brownsville was one of the poorest and most violent neighborhoods in the Borough. It was said to be the birthplace of Murder, Inc. We all lived in this harsh environment, but what was most memorable about Teddy was not his basketball skills, but his genuine concern for others. He was caring and kind and took on the role of protecting the most vulnerable in this menacing neighborhood.

One hot summer day, as I hung out in front of the poolroom, two large men began harassing Benny, a sweet, harmless 30-year-old guy. Benny appeared quite imposing, at about 6-foot, 220 pounds, but he was neurologically impaired. His speech and movements were awkward, but not so severe as to reveal his disability.

Seemingly, for no other reason but abject cruelty, the two unfamiliar bullies from outside the neighborhood were terrorizing Benny and making him cry. They continued to escalate their brutality by seeing how hard they could punch Benny in the stomach. The more Benny cried, the more the men laughed and punched him some more. Suddenly, from nowhere, it seemed, Teddy appeared. He moved as if he was flying through the air. The bullies never knew what hit them. In a flash of time and space, the two men were sprawled on the concrete sidewalk, their faces covered with blood. Teddy put his arm around Benny and wiped away his tears.

A few years later, I learned Teddy fell to his death while working at the Brooklyn Navy Yard. I will never forget him. I am sure he not only inspired me with his kindness and courage in looking after the less fortunate, but many others who were lucky enough to know him.

John Beard

In the early 1970s, I was working toward the completion of my doctorate in psychology and took a job at Manhattan State Psychiatric Center. The state hospital consisted of three foreboding twelve-story buildings, strategically placed on Ward's Island, isolated, surrounded by the East and Harlem Rivers. Built like a prison, it was less than a mile from the East Side of Manhattan, but light-years away. When you crossed the footbridge from Manhattan to the island, it was like walking back in time.

They put me to work in the Kirby Building on 6B, the female ward. Most of the women were longtime residents of the state hospital and victims of the regressive policy of locking away people with psychiatric disorders. The few young patients received most of the attention, the older ones, resigned and institutionalized, sat sullenly in the day room.

An ugly dark green paint covered the walls of the hospital ward. Rows of small box spring beds and wooden chairs were the only furniture except for two round tables in the day room. Dull lighting added to the misery. It was cold and stark.

The policy at the time was to push patients back into the community. Called humane, it resulted in discharging a wave of patients into dreadful single room occupancy hotels with little support and no hope. Isolated in their rooms, the patients had no place to go and nothing to do. I realized the best thing I could do for my patients would be to help them find a decent place to live.

One day in 1974, I visited Fountain House. I wasn't sure exactly what it was, but I'd heard it had an apartment program for psychiatric patients. I was awestruck from the first moment I walked through the door of the building on West 47th Street. Fountain House was remarkably beautiful. The furnishings, the architecture, the rugs, the artwork, all of it reminded me of a private university club, but the members were severely disabled psychiatric patients. These were the very same people I left back on Ward's Island; only here they were animated, interacting, and productive. I learned quickly that the proper terminology was members, not patients. In the greeting area, a member introduced himself and said he would be acting as our tour guide. We first took the elevator down to the dining room and the kitchen area, where the member showed me a well-equipped commercial kitchen and a large, cheery dining room buzzing with activity. Here, one social worker and about ten members were preparing lunch for the other members and the staff. The members were cooking, cleaning, talking, and even laughing.

Amazingly, the very same people with diagnoses of schizophrenia who had been sitting around the ward lost and defeated now appeared energized and productive. In the clerical unit, members answered the phones, typed letters, and prepared a daily newsletter. In the education and research unit, members kept data on attendance, hospitalizations, and employment placement.

The methodology of Fountain House was simple, yet brilliant. The facility was a place where they could socialize, though mostly in the evenings and weekends. During working hours, members contributed by helping to run Fountain House. The members, former institutionalized patients, felt needed and appreciated once again. The members honed their skills with the help of social workers and rehabilitation counselors, which made them more confident and productive. When they were ready, the members would work part-time at companies like American Express, Becton & Dickinson, and Sears. In the evening, the members would return to Fountain House, hang out at the snack bar and talk about their day's work. At night, they would go home to the apartments they shared with another member and leased by Fountain House.

Fountain House is a remarkable place that has transformed the lives of so many of society's most unwanted. I went to work there in 1976 as Director of their first National Institute of Mental Health grant to train mental health centers around the country in the Fountain House methodology. There are now Clubhouse Programs nationwide and internationally as well.

John Beard was the architect of this brilliant yet common sense approach to helping people with severe mental illness. A social worker by training, he was set on a path of finding a better way to help the mentally ill as a result of his own father's psychiatric illness. Fresh out of graduate school in the early 1950s, Beard worked in a state psychiatric hospital in Detroit, Michigan. He took groups of patients off the ward to baseball games at Tiger Stadium and to restaurants in downtown Detroit. Beard then called on a couple of companies in Detroit and asked for an entry-level job. He explained that he would train two patients to do the job. He promised that the work would get done every day, if not by the patient, then by himself. Open-minded companies embraced the concept. The program would help them fill positions with high turnover and high absenteeism, plus the work was guaranteed. Soon, chronically ill psychiatric patients were working successfully in downtown Detroit.

Beard came to Fountain House in 1955. He put groups of members and staff together on essential projects. The more the members were depended upon for their work and assistance, the healthier they became. The less they were treated as patients, the less they acted like patients. In his 20 plus years at Fountain House, Beard saw his ideas grow into an internationally renowned psychiatric rehabilitation program that has become the model for appropriate care.

John Beard was like no one in the mental health field I had ever known. He was transformative, charismatic, rebellious, and with his keen intelligence, attracted a wealthy and powerful board of directors. He enticed leaders from Wall Street and business to past presidents of Harvard to serve on the board. John won their hearts and minds by passionately conveying his ideas for changing the way we treat the mentally ill and restoring their dignity. The board raised private funds that enabled Beard to develop innovative programs that insurance companies and government agencies refused to fund.

The results became clear as more and more patients diagnosed with schizophrenia succeeded in their jobs. Beard's program demonstrated that seriously ill psychiatric patients could successfully live and work in the community with adequate support. While the mainstream focused on treating symptoms, Beard focused on the predominately healthy person who had been overwhelmed by the consequences of the illness. Beard's mission was to build the best possible rehabilitation program and then use it as a model to transform the way psychiatric patients were treated around the world. He succeeded!

Beard could have succeeded at anything and made loads of money, but instead, he reached out to society's most discarded and alienated and helped them build a life in the community. John was an exceptional moral leader and innovator in the care of the mentally ill. He was also a great teacher. He inspired me and had a profound influence on my work. John Beard died in 1982, but Fountain House lives on.

* * *

Who we are and who we will become is a study in progress. As long as we are open to new learning, we can continue to grow and evolve. Learning from role models, engaging in self-analysis, and an interest in ethical problem solving can all lead to moral growth. Moral integrity rests on the willingness to accept personal responsibility and the desire to examine one's behavior honestly.

Why Be Moral?

It is not easy being moral. It's not as simple as espousing an opinion, signing a petition, or making a donation. Being moral is not whether you're liberal or conservative, or what your passionate views may be on abortion, human rights, or the environment. We can all be high and mighty in our social commentary on world affairs, but what counts is the moral climate in our universe—our family, friends, and coworkers. Morality is intimate and personal. It is the personal moral issues that have profound influences on our relationships. We judge our moral conduct by whether there are consequences to others as a result of our behavior. Often, our honorable actions involve personal sacrifices to benefit the lives of others.

The vast majority of us are not in a position to elevate the moral landscape of our country, but we do have power. We can use the power of the Presidency as it relates to our family, our work, and our community. These personal moral issues have profound influences on our relationships and our well-being. Our moral conduct is what counts when we have a direct impact on people's lives. Elite moral conduct almost always involves a cost of time, energy, or resources employed to elevate the life of another: Who stands with the vulnerable, the target of the bully at work? Who sacrifices personal pleasures for the welfare of other family members?

Let's say you come across a man lying in the street, apparently hit by a car. Blood is pumping from the man's carotid artery. The poor man is in agony, blood is covering his face, and pooling onto the street. You immediately apply direct pressure while screaming for someone to call 911. The man's blood has splattered over your arms and face as you tend to him. His blood is in your hair. You can feel it trickling down your neck, and believe you can taste it. A chilling thought hits you that maybe you've been exposed to some infectious disease.

Or consider another scenario where the idea of infection strikes you as you approach the bleeding victim, and you decide to keep walking and leave it to some other passerby to help him.

* * *

One way of profiling elite moral conduct is by examining its polar opposite, the psychopath: Think about what it would be like to take wild risks and not feel any apprehension or worry. So confident and sure of yourself, you race ahead without any fear of failure. Now imagine you have no problem with lying or breaking the rules because "everyone does it." Besides, you're entitled.

And, you have this charismatic gift. You can charm and seduce just about anyone. You use this gift to manipulate people, getting what you want, and then walking away without a care. You don't worry about slipping up, and you don't feel even a tinge of guilt. You're smarter than just about anybody else, and you're going to get it all. The psychopath stalks his prey, manipulates his victims, and feels no remorse. His motives are sex, money, and power.

Buddy Jacobson personified this profile perfectly. He was intelligent, charming, cunning, and fearless, Jacobson compulsively pursued young women, money, and power. In the 1960s, he used illegal drugs to become the most successful thoroughbred trainer in the country.

He became bored with his success, stole money from his owners, left his wife and children to begin his relentless pursuit of beautiful young women. Jacobson purchased a ski resort in Vermont and apartment buildings on the East Side of Manhattan with the sole goal of seducing beautiful young women. He electronically bugged all thirty apartments in his apartment building, and only rented to female flight attendants and models. Driven by compulsive lust, he had to have a different young woman each night and then discarded them as he did his horses. Jacobson was ruggedly handsome and charming, enabling him to seduce the beautiful young model Melanie Cain and build a modeling agency on her stardom.

This psychopath eventually self-destructed when he murdered his rival for Melanie Cain. Anthony Hayden-Guest documented Jacobson's unbelievably successful and debased sociopathic life in his book *Bad Dreams*.

Ted Bundy, the infamous serial murderer, sought the ultimate power. What makes psychopaths such dangerous predators is that initially, they appear to be acting to benefit others. Their stealth enables them to mislead and devour their prey.

A former police officer, author Ann Rule first met Ted Bundy in 1971 when he was 24 and a senior at the University of Washington. Bundy, the horrific serial murderer, brutally killed and tortured anywhere from 30 to 60 women in the 1970s. Rule sat next to him at the Seattle Crisis Clinic, where they worked together, taking calls from those in despair contemplating suicide. Rule described Bundy's conversations with callers as caring, sincere, and reassuring. In her book, *The Stranger Beside Me*, she describes Bundy as follows:

"Ted was like a knight in shining armor. He was brilliant, a student of distinction, witty, glib, and persuasive. He favored French cuisine, good white wine, and gourmet cooking. A bright young man on his way up who might well have been Governor of Washington. He was one of those rare people who listened with full attention, who evince a genuine caring by their very stance. You could tell things to Ted that you might never tell anyone else."

We all know what happened to Ted Bundy, who escaped from jail twice, committing more murders and assaults before his capture and eventual execution at Florida State Prison. In time, the psychopath implodes. Their extreme narcissism and greed eventually incinerate them. Blinded by entitlement, driven by compulsions (e.g., Harvey Weinstein and Jeffrey Epstein), they self-destruct. Sadly, they leave too many victims in their wake.

Psychopathy—sociopathy, anti-social personality—represents the absence of morality. The psychopath displays moral behavior at its most debased and depraved. Ethical moral behavior is characterized by actions based on principled integrity, regardless of the consequences to the self. In contrast, actions that are in one's self-interest, despite the damage done to others, define psychopathy.

* * *

"Only a life lived for others is a life worthwhile."
~Albert Einstein

If you want to feel better about yourself, do something beneficial for someone else.

Elite moral behavior is not free, but the seeds you sow will reap rewards. The genuine appreciation one receives for helping others is a tonic for the soul. It makes life sweeter and more purposeful. It elevates self-worth and makes self-acceptance more acceptable.

Morally elite individuals are those who sacrifice their own needs and wants to pursue a course of conduct intended to benefit the lives of others. Many individuals live their lives with honor. Their worthy deeds are appreciated by those they touch, but mostly escape public recognition. An elite moral act that enhances the life of one person is qualitatively no different than conduct that betters the lives of thousands.

If you risk your life to rescue one person from a burning building, it is no less worthy than if you save a thousand.

Elite moral conduct is an achievement that is on par with any great discovery. It moves society forward by lifting our collective character. It elevates people and inspires them, helping to advance civilization. Don't bother asking a dedicated scientist who strives to develop a life-saving vaccine whether all his sacrifices are worth it. There is inherent meaningfulness in the pursuit of excellence; these dedicated individuals feel compelled to do their work. The same is true for a transcendent moral act. The act is intrinsically rewarding, and the moral leader has no choice. Their drive for selfless achievement is part of their moral fabric.

Making sacrifices of one's time, energy, and resources to facilitate another's growth, safety, and peace of mind is an avenue open to all of us. You may not think about the following examples as being in the elite category, but think again how you'd feel if you were on the receiving end: Giving assistance to an elderly neighbor, coming to the aid of a child in danger, providing "warmth" to someone left out in the "cold." This demonstration of elite moral conduct elevates the lives of members of our community and shows us the meaning of ethical leadership. We all have the capacity and the opportunity to be moral leaders.

Elite moral conduct has a spiritual element, a "lightness of being," and is a path to inner peace. Elite moral conduct doesn't mean you must relinquish pleasure. On the contrary, when you feel truly worthy, your pleasure is enhanced. So, when we ask, "Why be moral?" we can say it is the right thing to do and is in our own best interest.

PART THREE

There is No Future in Staying the Same

There is No Future in Staying the Same

Opening yourself to new learning and the flexibility to adapt is essential for growth, success, and survival. Being closed and rigid during changing times puts your future in peril. Openness to new learning implies the ability to alter one's views and behaviors based on different information or changed circumstances. There truly is no future in staying the same.

Admittedly, change is difficult, but remaining the same is a losing proposition. I don't mean voluntary change, like, "I'm moving to New Jersey to be close to my children." That's easy to adapt ourselves to, but we resist forced change that comes upon us, often unexpectedly. Nevertheless, our development from interacting with our environment demands it. Mess up the transition from diapers to the toilet, and you're in big trouble.

Our world is constantly shifting as we strive to find a place for ourselves. Technology, economic cycles, or politics can impact us, and suddenly we've lost our job. The shifting state of the economy over the past decade has eliminated many good jobs in steel, coal, and manufacturing sectors. Technology rapidly changed our lives. If you don't have a smartphone, computer, and Internet access today, you're on dinosaur time.

Individually, our world continually changes as we transition from children to adults. Major steps, like leaving home, starting a career, becoming a parent, and aging, has its hurdles. To thrive, we have to figure out what is in our best interest and adapt accordingly.

The more resistant we are to change, striving to avoid it, the more vulnerable we become. Our survival depends on our ability to recognize the need for change before it's too late. In the 1930s in Germany, many Jews saw incremental evidence of animus and terror but held on in denial. Germany was their home, after all. Their businesses and families were there, and too many Jews ignored the early warning signs and paid the price with their lives. They did not act in their best interest.

Our resistance to change, holding on to the past, is motivated by fear and entrenchment. Its accomplice is denial. Denial is the dysfunctional way of dealing with reality. Denial, a partly conscious process, blinds us to what we don't want to see. Denial distorts the truth. We resist change because we are fearful we may not be up to the task. We resent the need to change, telling ourselves, "This is who I am and what I do."

Denial is the irrational and self-destructive attempt to stay the same, and hope the problem goes away. When your ship is sinking, you can't keep doing things the same old way. Whatever the issue may be—health, career, or relationship issues—at some point, the problem is no longer the problem. The problem is one's inability to adjust to a changed reality.

You've heard it said that "Insanity is doing the same thing over and over again and expecting different results." Whether Albert Einstein said it or not, it's an apt definition for using denial as a form of magical thinking.

Charles Darwin (1809–1882), best known for his contribution to the science of evolution, emphasized the need to adapt to a changing world. Darwin wrote: "It is not the most intelligent of the species that survive, it is not the strongest that survive, the species that survive is the one best able to adapt and adjust to the changing environment that one finds themselves in."

And while our environment demands adaptation, we can

say the same about our inner world. Self-appraisal is crucial in capitalizing on our strengths and mitigating our weaknesses. Self-knowledge aids us in overcoming the roadblocks, the ebbs and flows of life.

Denial works for a while to avoid the pain of change until it doesn't. The ability to adjust to changing circumstances and the new reality is an actual test of our mental health. Mental illness and reality are not highly correlated. *AIYOBI* requires an accurate perception of reality and an accurate appraisal of ourselves.

Life can throw us a curveball, or worse, kick us in the stomach, at any age. That being said, we can identify three stages of life that are fraught with the need for change. The transition from adolescence to adulthood, the career and family challenges of midlife, and the stage of aging and loss.

Adolescence to Adulthood

The transition from adolescence to adulthood is one of life's most difficult bridges to cross. A myriad of challenges and demands confront this age group, and often in a totally new environment. There is a need for adjustments and adaptations in most areas of the individual's life during this transition period. The leap from dependent child to self-reliance is dramatically steep and can be an intensely stressful period. We tend to overlook this reality, fooled by youthful exuberance, imagined invulnerability, and hidden turmoil.

Let's consider the hurdles faced by a young person going off to college. Certainly, going off to work has significant challenges, but for now, we'll focus on the college experience. Perhaps it begins like this: "Kid, these are going to be the best years of your life. You'd better enjoy it before you face the real world." Some young people may indeed find college to be the best years of their lives, but for others, who are unprepared to go off on their own, it's the very worst time of their lives. Feelings of failure, alienation, anxiety, and despair fill their days.

"A mind is a place of its own, in it you can make a hell out of heaven, or a heaven out of hell."
~ John Milton, Paradise Lost

Grim statistics illustrate the stress associated with this period of life. Accidents, suicides, and homicides account for

74% of all deaths for young adults ages 14 to 24, according to 2017 data from the National Institute of Health (NIH).

Accidents - 40.6%
Suicides - 19.2%
Homicides - 14.4%
Cancer - 5.1%
Heart Disease - 2.9%

How many of the accidents, suicides, and homicides are marked by a failure to adjust, emotional distress, and self-sabotage? Unprepared for the challenge and unable to ask for help, many young people become victims of self-destructive behavior. This period can test one's mental health and the ability to adapt to changing circumstances.

Essentially, good mental health and the ability to adapt are the same. Further evidence of the stress related to this transition is reflected in the following National Institute of Mental Health (NIMH) data. Young adults, ages 18–25, have the highest prevalence of mental illness than any other age group.

2017 Data NIMH

Any Mental Illness	Serious Mental Illness
AGES: 18–25 — 25.8%	7.5%
26–49 — 22.2%	5.6%
50+ — 13.8%	2.7%

Increased stress always leads to an increase in symptomology for those who are vulnerable. Why is this time of life so difficult and painful for some, while others call it the best time of their lives? Many interacting factors account for it. For illustration purposes, let's follow a mythical 18-year-old male, who one day is living at home, and two months later, in college, finds everything has changed.

Here, all alone! Where do you fit in? Who seems interested in you? The hall appears to be filled with tall, good-looking dudes. Everybody seems to know each other. Academically, the work is much harder, and you can't just rely on class notes anymore. There is a need to read more, work independently, there are papers due, homework, and tests coming up. And you're way behind!

How do you manage your time and what you do when there's

no one there watching over you? There are alcohol and drugs, crazy parties, and sex. It's all out there.

Alone and feeling like an outcast. Have some more alcohol that will help. You find the texts boring and fall behind in your classes—play video games instead. No one seems to like you. You're staying in your room, alone, anxious, depressed. You just don't have the will to get things right. And then, thoughts of suicide fill your head.

This time of life delivers the sternest test of our mental health and our ability to *AIYOBI*. Discipline, the ability to delay gratification necessary for everything short of eating, drinking, and video games, is severely tested. The college environment produces the most stringent test of our ability to work for future goals. Do you party and play video games, or do you establish a work ethic?

This challenging time is when many serious mental health issues emerge, including identity problems, self-injury, schizophrenia, and suicide. Suicide is the second leading cause of death in this age group. The young are particularly vulnerable to suicide because their despair seems like it will last forever. They don't have the benefit of experience to realize that this episode will pass. The ebbs and flows of life are not part of their history.

What then differentiates those who flourish from those that are defeated? For the most part, with positive self-esteem and proper preparation, almost anything can be accomplished. The problem is self-esteem and preparation can't be purchased online. Instead, success depends upon the ubiquitous equation of G x E — Genes times Environment, which for most of us, means our parents. To a large degree, our parental environment determines how well prepared we are to meet the challenges of this stage of life.

Since our parents provide only 50% of our genetic make-up, they only contribute a portion of the equation. Nor do they account for the uniqueness factor, that magical element that gives us wings. This uniqueness could be a special talent, athletics, brilliance, or grace. A special attribute goes a long way in winning over the approval of others and quelling the demons that lurk inside our heads.

Self Esteem and Discipline

Every single thing about us, from our personality, to how fast we run, to how we value ourselves, is a function of our genes interacting with our environment. Our uniqueness, that exquisite element that truly expresses who we are, is the outcome of that volatile equation.

Our early years provide the foundation, and over time we shape our self-esteem and discipline. From conception, our neurobiology interfacing with our early life experience is the engineering of our unique "wiring." This wiring establishes neural pathways that shape our feelings, moods, and attitudes. Since our parents provide half our genes and create our home environment, they hold a lot of weight in the equation of who we are and how we value ourselves.

When we are young, parents are Godlike; they create the only universe we know. It can be a beautiful, nurturing, wise universe or a very dark and toxic one. We cherish good parenting for life. It prepares us for a stimulating and enjoyable life journey. On the dark side, toxic parenting leaves wounds that never truly heal.

Feeling worthwhile—valuing ourselves—is fundamental to self-discipline and *AIYOBI*. Why exert discipline and hard work to improve yourself if you're not worth it? Why delay gratification and give up the easy, quick fix when there is no future?

Good self-esteem is a work of art created by a loving parent when developed early in life. Parents help shape it during the everyday living experiences of the child, where opportunities for success evoke joy, growth, and self-confidence.

Modeling also plays an important role in a child's development. Parents with good self-worth transmit it to the child through observation and assimilation. The parents' behavior, demeanor, and feelings of competence are imperceptibly absorbed. They become the child's road map. The child thinks, "If my parents are worthy, I must be as well."

Developing good self-esteem in one's child requires thoughtful attention to that goal. Self-respect develops in increments over time. And all the effort, all the sacrifice pays off with the bliss of a child at peace with itself. Parents can either compensate for a child's vulnerabilities or exacerbate them. You can't change biology, but you can alter the environment. Experiencing things together and providing praise and corrective feedback leads to mastery and self-reliance. Wise parents encourage constitutionally timid children to approach new situations. They walk hand in hand, slowly, patiently, triumphantly overcoming the fear. It is a delicate balance of exposure and support until the child learns to feel secure.

Those children biologically predisposed to impulsivity, risk-taking, and aggressiveness offer a different challenge. How do we help these children gain thoughtful self-control prior to action? Observing and working with the child in play and social situations provide opportunities for corrective feedback. Children learn best when the guidance is provided at the moment in time. Specific feedback given with patience and kindness is likely to be internalized. Parental tone and demeanor influence the child more than the parent's words.

Punishing a child teaches nothing but who is in charge. Its consequence, submission perhaps, resentment for sure, and a lesson in primitive moral conduct of Might Makes Right. The thoughtful parent discusses the issues intending to impart wisdom. The thoughtless and the autocrat resort to penalization.

In a healthy environment, children learn that work and play can be the same. Work is valued as an accomplishment and not viewed as a burden or something to be avoided. Daily chores and homework reinforce the value of work.

Preparation is the foundation of success and is the outgrowth of discipline. When prepared for college, you understand before you ever get there that the course work will demand much more independent study than high school. You're mature enough to regulate your time and energy to meet your responsibilities in your role as a student. With good self-esteem, you embrace the new social environment.

You don't worry about finding friends. When you value yourself, people find you attractive.

Good self-esteem without discipline is often the outcome of well-intentioned, overly indulgent parents. One way to unwittingly obstruct a child's growth is to be overly indulgent. The parental goal is to protect the child and pave the way for them, but going overboard often results in a child with poor discipline who is unprepared for the challenges ahead. When the parent is the child's blocking back, they clear the path but undermine growth, maturity, and self-reliance. Overindulgence can also be a precursor to narcissism and a sense of entitlement. Wise judgment yields a proper balance between loving encouragement and accountability.

Self-esteem can be tenuous, particularly in young people. When good discipline is absent, failure is the likely outcome. Even with a good sense of self-worth, failure erodes self-confidence. All the parental overprotection does not serve the child well in their tango with the real world.

Discipline without love is the immoral display of power over the child, establishing obedience with intimidation, threats, and punishment. The child is compliant and well-disciplined as long as the dictator rules. At work or college, once liberated from the bully's dominance, discipline craters.

This type of parental discipline won't internalize the values of work and building for the future. Instead, it creates a dislike for authority figures.

Pete had the potential to soar like an eagle. He was smart, strong, could run like the wind, and was the best player on his high school football team. Pete's life lessons from his mean-spirited father came with a hard slap on the head, a metal buckle to his back, and vile attacks on his intelligence and manhood.

Pete lost his athletic scholarship in his first year at college. Betrayed by his father, authority figures became the enemy, and he couldn't trust his coaches and teachers. He wasn't prepared, failed his classes, and didn't show up on time for practice.

I met Pete when he was a patient on the brain injury unit. He suffered a depressed skull fracture after being hit on the head with a tire iron in a parking lot brawl outside a bar. A chronic alcoholic, he battled the demons of his father's sins with vodka.

* * *

When parents fail, when the glorious gifts of discipline and self love are absent, suffering inevitably follows. Developing discipline and learning to value oneself becomes a life long challenge. If one is fortunate, a mentor, perhaps a teacher, can become a role model and inspire growth and discipline. In such a case, the kindness of others can save the day for the victim of toxic parenting. A true friend, someone who believes in you and values you, can make a world of difference.

AIYOBI is not only a product of self-esteem and discipline but also paradoxically the path to achieving it. Achievement builds improved self-esteem. When we successfully accomplish something, we feel good about ourselves. Achievement is an elixir that instills a sense of competence and well being.

Here's the conundrum: Improved self-esteem grows from accomplishment, which in turn is built on discipline. If you are lacking in discipline, how do you achieve anything? You can't change how you feel by bemoaning your fate. So, act as if you love yourself even if you don't feel it. Try becoming the loving parent to yourself that you would like to be to your child. Small positive self-enhancing actions build on one another incrementally. There is a momentum to achievement; its rewards fuel further advances.

If you don't feel worthy, act like you do. It's a grind, I know. There is no magic pill. It means giving up the chocolate donut and cleaning the house. A good therapist's primary goal is to win over the trust of the patient, become their ally, and then influence them to *AIYOBI*. If we can listen to our voice of reason, we can become our best ally.

Midlife

Paraphrasing Darwin, it's not the smartest or the strongest that thrive but those best able to adapt to changing circumstances. Marriage, children, money/career, relocation, the unexpected, all call upon our ability to adjust and adapt to new challenges.

When confronted with the need to change, stress is its cohort, but growth is its prize. Those who are well adjusted and adapt well defuse the tension gracefully. A gain in self-confidence and competence is their reward. Unable to adapt, the stress wears you down.

Clarifying the concepts of adapt and adjust, we adapt to changing circumstances by adjusting our behavior and expectations. A well-adjusted individual encounters new situations with openness to new learning. For example, in my work as the Director of the Head Injury Rehabilitation Center, the strongest predictor of a patient's adaptation following brain injury of similar magnitude was how well adjusted the individual was before their injury.

Marriage

Why do people marry? There are many reasons, but I'm not sure the participants know why at the time. Until recently, the shortest marriage I knew of lasted one night. The bride, my wife's friend, called the next morning and said it was all a big mistake. A few years later, a friend who worked at a beach resort told me about this poor bride's experience. After their stunning wedding on the ocean's edge, the happy couple retreated to their honeymoon suite. It was 2:00 a.m. when the groom pushed his naked bride into the hallway and locked the door. Frantic and nude, she knocked on doors until a "good Samaritan," a single young male, took her in for the night.

People reveal who they are over time, although sometimes it takes a very long time. But, as Einstein said, time is relative. How do you adjust when the honeymoon is over? Make sure you set boundaries at the beginning. Establish how you want to be treated early in the relationship. When maltreatment goes unchecked, it swells and erodes the relationship. If the abuse continues, it becomes the norm and is then very difficult to change.

Some couples live, work, and sleep together 24/7. Others seem to live truly separate lives. Some maintain strong sexual desire for their partners, while others completely lose interest and either abstain or look elsewhere. Values, children, and shared finances all come into play in the day-to-day relationship, making it one of the most challenging partnerships imaginable. When and how it all gets worked out is a mystery. Nevertheless, some fundamental principles hold true. Marriage is not about sex, and when the lust fades, who is in the foxhole with you? Here are three simple axioms to keep in mind:

1. Do they have your back?
2. Are they honest and trustworthy?
3. Are they a good person with good moral values?

Sam, a patient of mine, in his mid-sixties, had the misfortune of developing one medical problem after another. He had been in and out of the hospital with neurological and kidney issues, when his wife of twenty years told him, "She didn't buy into this." I never met his wife Karen but learned it was Sam's second marriage, and she was quite a bit younger than he was.

During his most recent hospitalization, Sam asked her to bring his favorite pajamas. Karen told him she didn't like going to the hospital, and he should wear whatever they gave him. The very next day, she called and told him she was moving out and going home to live with her mother. There was no future being his caretaker, she said, informing him she wanted out of the marriage and was meeting with her lawyer.

Resigned, Sam told me all of this with little emotion. Oh, he was hurt, but not that surprised. I asked him earnestly, "Sam, tell me, really, what did you see in her?" He smiled and said, "She had the most beautiful ass and legs you've ever seen."

* * *

What do you do when you find out your spouse is having an affair? Laura, a 42-year-old mother of two, knew her husband Tom was unfaithful. He acted guilty when he came home from work, much too accommodating, too nice. There were times when his clothing had the faint scent of strange perfume. Tom and a female coworker occasionally traveled together on business trips, and Laura suspected they were having an affair.

When convinced he was unfaithful, she confronted him. Tom admitted it and seemed almost relieved to get it out in the open. He told her it was just sex, and the other woman didn't mean anything to him. He said it was over, apologized profusely, and promised it wouldn't happen again.

Laura felt betrayed. She was so angry she could hardly stand to be in the same room with him, feeling like she was living with the enemy. It wasn't just the sex, but all the lies he had told her. His adultery had broken the bond of honesty they had with one another. Laura's immediate reaction was purely emotional. Enraged and humiliated, she wanted out of the marriage because she just couldn't trust him anymore.

When she came to see me a couple of weeks later, her anger had dissipated somewhat, but she still felt betrayed and didn't know what to do. She was thinking about divorce but wasn't sure that was the right thing to do.

After a few sessions, I learned that Tom was a loving parent and generally a good person. Laura related that she always believed she could trust him until this latest mess. She said he had always been supportive, and she had thought of him as her best friend.

Here were my questions to Laura: Does his sexual indiscretion overrule everything else about him? On balance, is this sufficient reason to end the marriage, or in the larger scheme of things, only a big bump in the road?

In time, over the next few months, when her wounded feelings began to heal, Laura was able to see things more clearly. She was able to put the episode in context, and her measured thoughts trumped emotion. Tom was a good man, and Laura stayed in the marriage. She realized that it was in everybody's best interest.

* * *

Financial independence is power, and when possible, both partners should share this power. Dependency, either financial or emotional, is the antecedent of control and resentment. It leads to an unhealthy imbalance in the relationship. When you're working and earning a living, you have strength. You don't have to be the victim of your partner's maltreatment. I used to share this primarily with young women, now everyone hears it and understands it.

When boundaries fail, the question becomes, "Should I stay, or should I go?" One's ultimate leverage has to be, "If you continue to treat me this way, I will leave you." And it should never be said as a bluff, the courage to leave must be there.

The day after Carol went missing, her husband called me angry and distraught, "Do you know where she is?" he asked.

"She said she was going to the dentist and never came home. What kind of bullshit ideas have you put in her head?" he screamed into the phone.

I didn't know where Carol was, but I wouldn't have told him if I did.

Carol, a fifty-year-old mother of three grown children, came to see me because of her painful marriage to Frank. She told me a story of thirty years of emotional and physical abuse. She felt trapped, she said, because Frank was "a good provider," and at times even "fun to be with." But there was a very steep price to pay.

Carol lived in constant fear, treading on eggshells whenever they were together, never knowing what might trigger Frank's explosions. He demeaned her in public, calling her stupid in front of their friends. When he hit her, he told her it was her fault for being such "a dumb bitch."

The first time I saw Carol, she cried through the entire session. Beaten into submission, she believed what Frank told her, that "She was too stupid to make it on her own." The pattern of abuse over three decades had worn her down, so maybe Frank was right, and she couldn't make it without him.

I found Carol to be an intelligent, competent person. She

didn't have any severe mental health problems except for her pathological relationship with Frank. When the children came, Carol had stopped working, and her priority became to keep the family together. In the process, she lost touch with her independence, and it slipped away over time.

The last time Frank hit her, she had been out with her girlfriends and came home a half-hour late. As she walked through the door, Frank struck her so hard he knocked her across the room. He was out of control, and she feared for her life. That was the last straw. She knew she couldn't live like this anymore and made an appointment to see me.

"I don't know what to do," she said. "Do I just walk away after thirty years?" I told her, even if she wanted to remain in the marriage, the only leverage she had was divorce. The ultimate ultimatum. Tell him, "Either you treat me decently, or I'm out of here and will take half of what is rightfully mine."

She tried, but she just couldn't do it. The thought of confronting Frank was too frightening. She believed he wouldn't care what she said; his face would redden, he'd ball up his fists, and call her every name under the sun.

Instead, Carol surreptitiously hired a lawyer, told Frank of her fictitious dental appointment, and never returned home. Sadly, it took thirty years for Carol to gather the strength and self-confidence to act in her own best interest.

* * *

Why have children? Once again, I'm not sure the participants know why. Most people underestimate the time, energy, and resources needed to raise children. Having kids dramatically alters our lives and tests our ability to adjust and adapt. Some observations:

• Parenting is a job of giving and sacrificing. Narcissists need not apply.

• If you don't have adequate resources, think again. Raising children is tough enough when resources are plentiful.

• It's hard work that often goes unappreciated, but when done right with genuine passion, the effort is joyful, and the prize is the universe.

Money

Money is not only the root of evil; it is the root of survival. For animals it is food and water, for us it is money. However, pursuing money beyond reason is shallow. When we use it to provide a better life for one's family, it is vital.

Money doesn't seem that important when we're young.

That's the time to chase one's dream. You can live the life of an artist when you're only responsible for yourself. But when a family is on the horizon, things change dramatically. How do you adapt when you find out how much money you need to live well? You can enjoy following your passion on your own and not obsess about money, but with children, you must have the financial resources to provide every opportunity for them.

Washington and Hollywood don't seem to understand that it's hard to dwell on global warming when these more immediate issues consume us:

- Finding a safe and peaceful place to live for you and your family.
- Having access to good health care.
- A good school system.
- Feeling secure and independent.

It's nice to be able to go to a hotel during a hurricane, rather than sleep on the floor in a shelter. The government is not the answer. Medicaid, food stamps, and subsidized housing offer a very meager existence.

The challenge then is how to make enough money to provide a safe and secure environment for your family? Once again, it is survival of the fittest. This may sound cold and harsh, but it is reality. When faced with such a challenge, we must utilize all the available tools for survival, including researching opportunities, education and training, relocation, and accurate self-appraisal. Our drive, resiliency, and the ability to adjust and adapt are severely tested during life-altering situations. Those best able to adjust and adapt to our ever-changing reality win their future.

Work is hard. Most of us are not working at our dream job. The reality of providing for our families is where we learn the hunt isn't always easy. Over the years, the most common complaints I've listened to were not about the work itself but poor treatment on the job. Workers feel unappreciated, stifled, unfairly criticized, yelled at, forced to play political games, having to kiss the boss's ass, underpaid, and passed over for promotions. These are the most familiar tales of woe.

Yes, people can be disappointing, and it's especially hurtful when they have leverage over you at work. You can turn the tables on them by remembering that EXPERTISE IS POWER. If you do your job better than anyone else, you're indispensable, and nobody is going to mess with you. If you are really good at what you do, your ticket is punched to go anywhere. If your present boss doesn't appreciate you, there will be many suitors waiting in the wings.

However, if you just think you're good, but you're not, then the problem is self-appraisal.

Money can also be a fool's game. Engaging in social comparisons with those who have a bigger house or faster car is the entertainment of idiots. Envy is the irrational response to someone you perceive as doing better than you. Likewise, using the size of your bank account as the basis of your self-esteem can leave you morally bankrupt. Driven by greed to pursue money recklessly leads to bad things happening in the form of self-destructive behavior.

What else does midlife throw at us? Is this it? Is this all there is? A midlife depression often lurks when things go wrong. Life is hard. There are divorce and illness, financial pressures, and unforeseen events.

COURAGE IS HAVING THE FORTITUDE NOT TO BE INTIMIDATED BY LIFE. WHEN YOU'RE ABLE TO ADAPT, YOU FEEL CAPABLE OF HANDLING WHAT LIFE THROWS AT YOU.

Old Age

What happened, how did I get here? I've battled demons in early life and had my mid-life problems, but adjusting and adapting to old age is by far the most difficult stage for me.

Old age is a feeling, not only marked by time but state of mind. Slowly, old age creeps upon us, bringing with it the tyranny of loss - loss of power, purpose, and belonging, but most painful is the loss of well-being. Most of us first feel old when we suffer some physical setback that is not transient but permanent. Hard reality hits us that we're in decline, a road we all unwillingly travel. Fearing the loss of one's physical or mental health is burdensome. You feel more vulnerable, fragile, and not as capable of handling life's obstacles.

Relentlessly, death comes knocking at our door. Our friends die, old family members fade away, and there is no one to call anymore.

Grief consumes us with the loss of a spouse, and there's no escape. We know it's coming for us. Every ache and pain could signal the beginning of the end. Illness is experienced differently in old age. Rather than thinking it's something to get well from, we fear it's never going to get better.

Old age is a brazen thief robbing us of part of our identity. I was always the person who helped others in a crisis.

Now I fear someone will have to help me. Once our work identity is gone, our culture devalues us and inundates us with drug and diaper commercials. Developers build self-contained communities to keep us out of sight and among our peers. Being old is not seen as "cool," and in most cases, young people don't want to hang out with us—unless, of course, you're Mick Jagger, then age doesn't matter.

The media tells us we're old with the news of the day, and the TV commercials advertise everything from walk-in bathtubs to stair-lift elevators. My mail isn't any better, providing me with a daily barrage of hearing aid offers and greetings from crematoriums.

Our politicians love to call their constituents ordinary people. A term they would never apply to themselves because time and age are apparently of no consequence to the powerful. The average age of U. S. Senators is nearly 62. And look at the age of the two 2020 presidential candidates and the Queen of England. Our shallow culture worships celebrity, and as Chris Rock once said, "Washington, D.C. is the Hollywood for ugly people."

Independence

In young adults, it's the transition, and in midlife, it's the battle. Old age's greatest threat is the loss of independence. The fear of loss of mobility is palpable. Becoming physically disabled or mentally incompetent is the shark in the water.

Losing financial freedom and burdening your family, or worse, relying on government assistance, is a close second. Sadly, this is not a problem that can be easily solved in this phase of life. Most of us don't have sufficient earning power in old age to make a difference in lifestyle.

Having insufficient funds in old age is not only a problem of the poor but the nearsighted with money. Once again, denial is the culprit and immediate gratification, the prize. "Why worry about tomorrow, spend it now."

Memory and Thinking

Dementia is an ugly word defining a decline in memory and thinking. The term is usually assigned to the elderly, though in past years has been used more indiscriminately. Dementia is an ill-chosen word that can refer to many different conditions. I prefer the term cognitive decline, which is more descriptive and less unworthy.

Alzheimer's disease, the most common and the most feared cause of cognitive decline in the elderly, is a vicious thief robbing us of our memory, causing us to lose our way by cutting the cords to reality. How often have you heard it said, or even said yourself?

I'm losing my memory. I'm worried that I can't remember things. I'd rather die than have Alzheimer's.

My work as a neuropsychologist has taught me the following: It's hard to measure our memory objectively. There are memory lapses that are part of being human. Misplacing things, walking into a room and forgetting why we went in there and forgetting people's names are all examples of normal forgetfulness. Recall usually declines with age, but remember at 75, we have a lot more stored up there than a 25-year-old. If plagued by worry about memory, get evaluated by a neuropsychologist.

Alzheimer's disease is not normal forgetting. It's a pathology where the usual first site of the attack is in the hippocampus of the brain. The hippocampus, about the size of a walnut, is essential for recording new memories, new learning, and continuous memory. If the hippocampus is completely damaged, we cannot recollect any of our new experiences. We have no continuous memory and live in a murky, momentary world where confusion, chaos, and alienation take hold.

New information not recorded in our brain is lost forever, typically an early symptom of the disease. If not recognized by the individual, family members will notice. There's no memory of recently shared experiences, so there's a tendency to repeat oneself and ask the same questions more than once. Alzheimer's timeline of progression varies, but as the disease ravages more and more of the brain, the person you knew vanishes.

Unfortunately, when it comes to memory and Alzheimer's disease, there is a lot of misinformation, and some of it is driven by greed. These are my observations from working in the field of neuropsychology for many years:

The current medications don't work, and the side effects typically outweigh any minimal, temporary benefits. As of 2019, the pharmaceutical companies have spent billions of dollars on research with no success to date.

There is no miracle food, vitamin, herb, or substance that improves memory. Eat a healthy diet, exercise, and beware of snake oil salesmen.

Forgetting because you're distracted or engaged in automatic behavior (putting your keys down) are not signs of Alzheimer's. Instead of memory exercises, stay involved in real activities of daily living like making a shopping list, preparing dinner, double-checking bills, and balancing the checkbook. Whatever the cause of memory deficits, developing compensatory tools early on can be helpful. For example, you might try the following:

- Start a daily log of activities and appointments.
- Start a diary to record the important events of the day.
- Put up a bulletin board in the kitchen listing appointments and projects as well as orientation information.
- Use tech-assisted devices such as a smartwatch for reminders to take medication and other responsibilities.
- Try not to fear the disease, but outwit it with compensatory tools.

The second most formidable enemy of our brain's memory and thinking is vascular disease, i.e., strokes. When our brain cells fail to get adequate blood supply, they become necrotic and die. Called ischemia, one's mental and physical losses are directly related to the areas of the brain affected. Vascular disease is profoundly different from Alzheimer's disease, and many strokes are preventable. The most ferocious enemy of our brain's health and our kidneys, for that matter, is chronic high blood pressure. Elevated BP damages blood vessels, which can lead to many different brain pathologies. Life taking hemorrhage strokes, bleeds into the brain, are often caused by chronic high BP.

In a condition called multi-infarct dementia, multiple small strokes cumulatively lead to severe cognitive decline. Again, the culprit is untreated high BP. The failure to monitor and get treatment for elevated BP is irrational. The emotion driving the irrational behavior is fear. Fear's disguise is denial: "I don't feel any symptoms, I feel fine, why should I start taking medication?" Yes, the medication can have unpleasant side effects, making the patient feel tired and listless. That's the price of staying alive and keeping all of your faculties.

Mortality

Nobody told me when I was young that this was all temporary. What was the point in overcoming all life threw at me if I am no more in the end? The realization that we're not going to be here much longer is oppressive. We always knew that day would come, but it becomes much more menacing as the time approaches. Somehow, we need to come to peace with this reality because you can't buy your way out. Some people have their faith to provide strength and inner peace. Those with the fire still burning fight death every step of the way.

As we approach the end, there are decisions to be made about treatment regimens, financial matters, and so much more. The most profound dilemma, in my opinion, weighs heavily and comes with no easy answer. After working with the chronically ill for many years, a doctor friend and I would lament there's nothing better than sudden death. What happens when suffering dwarfs pleasure? When it takes a team of workers to care for us, and all control is virtually gone? Is life worth living if we're languishing in a nursing home?

Most of us don't have good options for the end game. Our beloved pets are better off because veterinarians assist them to their final rest. Physician-assisted euthanasia is available in a few states but has significant drawbacks. Is suicide an acceptable way to end one's life?

I believe we have the moral right to let go in old age, but it gets much harder from there, with tough decisions to be made. You can't wait too long, and you need to be fit enough because you're on your own. Legally, no one can help you. How do we work it out with our loved ones? Do we tell them of our plans before and ask for their acceptance? Or, do we keep it secret and explain later with a note? Where do we do it? Certainly, not in our home, but where? How do we do it? Pills are uncertain, a gun, hanging, perhaps a long alcohol abetted swim in the ocean? Suicide is not wrong in old age; it is just very difficult.

A major theme of this book has been adapting and adjusting to the reality we find ourselves in. I believe it is empowering to have a choice whatever our stage of life. My first choice would be to go with the same kindness afforded my Golden Retrievers. Hopefully, that will be an option in the future, but certainly not in my lifetime. Perhaps, I'll take to the sea. I'll have a few drinks and start swimming. I'm not sure. Will I have the courage, the physical strength, or the conviction to leave my wife behind? Like everything else in life, the hardest part is execution.

The Tonic

Once we accept the reality that we're old, it is no longer threatening. Acceptance is the prelude to adjustment and adaptation—what we lose in foot speed; we compensate with wisdom. This is the time to give. It is the opportunity to use our wisdom to benefit the lives of others.

Engagement

The loss of purpose and belonging are much more painful than one's age. Ask any thirty-five year old professional athlete who has been cut from their team about the losses they suffer. Once more in life, we need to adapt. The absolute key to adapting to this stage of life is ENGAGEMENT. I can't stress this enough, involvement is essential, most beneficially, when we are interacting with others. Pain specialists will tell you that the two most important psychological factors in the experience of pain are our mood and what we are ATTENDING TO. Sitting at home, paying attention to every ache, and mental and physical pain is debilitating at any age. As the 19th-century psychologist and philosopher William James said, "My experience is what I agree to attend to."

Engagement is the act that knows no age barriers. It liberates us from the inner demons that take hold in times of dread. Keep working, volunteer, enroll in college courses, and focus your attention on something that takes you outside yourself. A passion, whatever it might be, is timeless. When we are involved with something meaningful, we transcend our personal woes.

Do you think you're too old? Look at the candidates in the 2020 campaign: Trump is 73, Biden 77, Bloomberg 77, and Sanders is 78. Maybe you can run for President. What do you think they would be doing if they weren't in the race? Sitting at home, feeling old and ruminating over their pain. Get in the race! Who says you can't start a new career? Feeling needed and productive is vital, and in our best interest regardless of our stage of life.

Love

It's never too late for love. Find someone to love. Your dog doesn't know how old you are, and he doesn't care. Love is timeless. Love has no age restrictions. It is an exquisite elixir for whatever ails you. Look for it, appreciate it, and keep the yearning alive. A few months ago, I asked my 74-year-old friend who has many medical problems, when he first felt old. He replied, "Why should I feel old? I have a 70-year-old girlfriend who is beautiful and who loves me."

We all can't find girlfriends, but we can find love. My

eighty- four-year-old friend brings his golden retriever to visit children in the hospital and he finds love every day. Help
someone in need, you'll find love and feel younger.

Define the Moment

Paradoxically, moments in time are timeless. When we are
deeply involved, we are ageless. If we remain in the moment,
we can have the eyes of a child. While the past may have re-
grets, and the future apprehensions, the moment is free to be
defined. Moments turn to minutes, and our pain becomes a
whisper. The most powerful attribute of old age is wisdom.
Use it to find peace and beauty. Enjoy the sunrise, the bird
in flight, and the wind against your face.

CPSIA information can be obtained
at www.ICGtesting.com
Printed in the USA
BVHW031219051120
592524BV00007B/737